Take It Off
and
Keep It Off

Anonymous

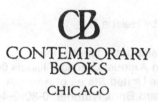

CONTEMPORARY
BOOKS
CHICAGO

Library of Congress Cataloging-in-Publication Data

Take it off and keep it off : based on the successful
    methods of Overeaters Anonymous / Anonymous.
        p.   cm.
      Bibliography: p.
      ISBN 0-8092-4493-4
      1. Reducing.   2. Reducing—Psychological
aspects.
RM222.T35   1989
613.2'5—dc20   89-33024
                                                  CIP

*To all those wonderful people who have supported me
through the years.*

*Special appreciation to Jerry and Bebe for their
continued encouragement.*

Published by Contemporary Books, Inc.
180 North Michigan Avenue, Chicago, Illinois 60601
Manufactured in the United States of America
International Standard Book Number: 0-8092-4493-4

The food plans discussed in this book are used as examples only; before starting any new food regimen, readers should consult a doctor or nutritionist. Also fundamental to the OA program are the 12 Steps of Recovery and the Twelve Traditions. Readers are encouraged to seek out the many good sources of information available on this subject, including those listed in the suggested reading list at the back of this book.

Contents

Contents

Introduction

I've gained and lost over one thousand pounds in my lifetime—fighting the battle of the bulge, bouncing on and off one diet or another. You name the diet, I've tried it. Most of these diets have helped for a short period of time, but I was never able to sustain a long-term weight loss.

As I look back over the years, many images come to mind regarding this "yo-yo" syndrome of losing and gaining the weight. In junior high school, I would open my nearly empty lunch box and see two tiny diet "wafers" wrapped in cellophane. It took about thirty seconds to finish them, and I was left with fierce stomach grumbles. By the time school let out at three o'clock, the local pizza vendor was serving his favorite customer—me.

My twenties were marked by many fad diets. The "water cure-all" promised me the body I'd always dreamed about. I starved myself and drank gallons of water. It was awkward walking down the street, because

I would have to run into coffee shops to use their facilities.

The "all-you-can-eat protein panacea" was next. What do you think I did with that one? I knew no limits. When I was given "permission" to eat all the protein I wanted to, I did just that. I'm only a little thing (5'4") and five pounds came on very quickly. This protein diet didn't work for me—I gained weight instead of losing it.

I had my blinders on when it came to quick weight loss and would follow anyone who promised me that I could be thin! But fad diets never worked for me. God only knows that I tested every new one that came out. With those regimens, I lost weight only to gain it right back again. They never taught me how to handle my new image or how to cope with real-life problems.

The final humiliation came in my late twenties, when I decided to visit a diet doctor. I took grueling train rides to get there and paid $40 a week for his magic potions. I trusted what he told me: "Take these drops before bed, and your appetite will be reduced—you'll lose weight." The only problem was that instead of diminishing my appetite, the drops made me an insomniac. While I was awake at night, I ran to the *refrigerator*. There's an added twist to this story. My medical guru was arrested five years later for fraud. (I could have made my own potions with a little water and food coloring.) I wonder how many other "gurus" are out there pedaling concoctions that are dangerous to our health!

When I was in my early twenties, my best friend was killed in an automobile accident, and all I could do was eat to numb the pain. Paradoxically, overeating also served as my greatest reward. When I landed my first job out of college, I treated myself to a fattening meal in the fanciest restaurant I could find.

Don't let these sad tales dismay you. I'm here to tell you *good* news. This lady who could never keep the weight off has kept fifty pounds off for sixteen years. To sustain my weight loss, I had to do lots of other things—such as learning to deal with my emotions and learning that I was not alone in my feelings or my overeating.

In retrospect, the pain of all my thwarted attempts to lose weight made me desperate enough to ultimately reach out for help. I had always been able to hide from myself how much weight I put on. But at age twenty-seven, this denial was broken while I was vacationing in Puerto Rico. In a glass cabana door at poolside, I caught a glimpse of myself wearing my mother's bathing suit. My thighs were enormous, and I felt as if I had "elephant legs." I was really fat! This awareness didn't stop me from popping chocolate candies in my mouth. However, I realized for the first time that I was sick, and that served as a turning point for me. When I got home, I joined a support group and was ready to listen to other people who seemed to have had some success in licking their food problem. They taught me how to eat sensibly and gave me the courage to explore the reasons for my overeating and understand my obsession about food.

Through talking with other people, I accepted the fact that overeating had served as a coping mechanism for me. I was inadequately equipped to handle my life, and food filled many gaps. It was my "best friend"— something I could turn to for comfort. It was my "lover"—keeping me company on those lonely Saturday nights. It was a "confidant"—I could isolate myself with it and close off the world when problems arose. Food was my buffer, and I consoled myself with it when life dealt me one of its blows.

A Little Bit About What I Ate to Take It Off

When I was reducing, I ate quite simply. While at home, I weighed my food on a small kitchen scale. This discipline helped me be honest with myself about what a normal portion was. You see, I had been eating for all the wrong reasons—loneliness, frustration, and so on. I was confused about the difference between healthy eating and using food to feed my emotional hunger.

When the weight began to melt away—and it did (on an average of two pounds a week)—I felt wonderful but frightened. A *sexy*, *alive*, and *visible* person was emerging, getting whistles from men as I walked down the street. For the first time in my life, I was slender for more than a month. (Only once before had I lost twenty-five pounds, and I gained it back within two weeks.) I felt very exposed—like one of those monkeys in a psychological experiment that has trouble eating because it was raised by a surrogate mother. I wanted to hide a lot because I didn't know how to handle all the attention I was getting. Thin is *not* well. I had always thought that if I just got down to "goal weight," everything would be OK. But that wasn't true! I began to realize what I had really been hungering for.

I hungered to feel cared about and loved.

I hungered to be part of the group, rather than feeling separate from it.

I hungered to be able to share myself more with people.

I hungered for self-love—to respect myself and do what was best for me.

I hungered to reach my potential in my career.

I hungered for acknowledgment from other people.

I hungered for the freedom to be myself and know that other people would accept the real me.

I hungered to let go of my judgments about myself and other people.

I hungered for a beautiful body—as I rightly deserved.

I didn't know how to handle these new awarenesses. I had never developed the tools for managing my life as a slender person.

The last five pounds were the toughest to lose and seemed to be cemented on me from birth. It took almost six months for that weight to drop off my body. But I needed this time to get used to me. I bought new clothes and learned to say thank you when someone gave me a compliment. I was facing the world for the first time as an attractive young woman.

When I finally reached my goal weight, I had to deal with a whole new set of problems. Could I take back the foods I had once loved? I had given up candy, cake, and ice cream, all of my "binge" foods, foods I couldn't stop eating after taking one bite. No one had the answers for me. I had to discover my own way of handling maintenance, which felt very disarming. There wasn't a prescribed way of eating anymore, and even my doctor didn't know what was right for me.

The secret to my long-term success is that I had a lot of help along the way. Through trial and error, and *not alone*, I found out what gourmet foods were OK to have and in what amounts. This involved a process of sharing my ups and downs with other people, which took several months. To get through it, I needed patience, patience, and more patience.

I worked out a new food plan with someone who had been maintaining her weight for a while. We tried one new food a week; anything more would have been unmanageable for me. My first egg roll was such a turn-on that I had to rush to call her after I finished it. It felt terrific knowing that I had a friend who would listen to my "food tales." I could also talk over my mistakes, which helped me to keep from pigging out when a food choice felt uncomfortable.

Today I eat everything within moderation—except the "binge" foods I mentioned before. Yes, I would love to eat lobster Newburg every night of the week, but at age forty-three, my body would take on rolls of fat in no time. And I still weigh my protein portion if I'm eating at home, which keeps me on the straight and narrow.

My food plan is flexible. It's all-purpose, designed for someone who goes everywhere and does everything. Whether I'm at a business luncheon or at a family dinner, it works for me.

I enjoy my meals. Ripe bananas have replaced rich cakes and ice cream. And a well-cooked artichoke is as delicious as a bag of french fries ever was. It was worth all the confusion and fear I experienced to acquire what I have today—a body that I'm proud of and a mind free from obsessions about food.

Imagine Being Slim

It's miraculous! For 5,760 days I've been slim. Through "thick and thin," I have remained faithful to a sane way of eating.

It hasn't always been easy, to put it mildly. I can remember being at an elaborate wedding where the meal was not served till 1:00 A.M. By the time it came, I wanted to eat everything in sight. But I didn't. What saved the night was making a phone call to a friend. She knew about my struggle with food and just listened while I raved. She reminded me about how bad I'd feel the next day if I overate. Making the call enabled me to go back to the table and eat a normal meal.

My own honeymoon in Mexico almost became a disaster when I came down with Montezuma's revenge. I have learned never to skip a meal, because I tend to want to eat twice as much during the next one. So while I lay uncomfortable in bed, my new husband had to fake some Spanish and bring me a roll and butter for dinner.

Excuses, excuses, and more excuses. I always found them when I wanted to eat. How can anyone control herself at a company dinner? Well I *did*, but it was tough. The main course was easy, because we were sitting around making small talk. But dessert was one of those do-it-yourself buffets, and my colleagues left the table to make their own ice cream sundaes. I couldn't bear sitting there alone, so I called a friend. She laughed when I told her, "The sundae almost seduced me." Her sweetness was better than any dessert ever tasted.

Just after I lost fifty-five pounds, I bought a white bikini and decided to treat myself to a Club Med vacation in Martinique. This trip was a test for me. Would I be able to resist those gourmet feasts far away from home? I was determined that this vacation would be different from all the rest and that I wouldn't indulge in the buffets. To accomplish this, I was prepared to do anything that was necessary.

I accomplished my goal because the food served became less important to me than the fun of the trip—walking along the beautiful beaches, going water skiing for the first time, and enjoying the exciting people I met. I was involved in the joy of living rather than the joy of food.

I wrote postcards each day to a friend, listing what I planned to eat. She didn't think I was crazy because she knew how hard it was for me to keep slender.

Praying helped, especially before I entered the dining room where the amazing buffet luncheon was served. The way I coped with this meal was to take only one serving of food. When the other vacationers went back for seconds and thirds, it was my cue to go for a walk on the beach.

I've learned to accept my limitations. Sitting at a table while other people are stuffing themselves is a setup for me, and if I'm not careful, I'll start overeating too. I *have choices*, and I keep this in mind all the time.

One summer, after months of slaving in the office, I decided on the spur of the moment that I needed a break. So I signed up for a cruise. Once I was on board, I noticed that everyone was talking about the midnight snack. They described it as an endless array of every kind of dessert you ever imagined. (Remember, desserts are my binge food.) Thank God, I realized that even looking at this gala spread would start me salivating, so I stayed as far away from it as possible. When the noshers made a mad dash to the snacking area at midnight, I danced up a storm on deck. Wouldn't you know that at breakfast, those passengers were groaning about how much they had eaten the night before. Not me; I felt terrific and free.

Two summers ago, my husband and I drove to Quebec and Montreal. The French Canadians are well known for their saucy delights. I knew that on this trip, my dinner meals would be richer than what I was accustomed to, so I decided to have simple breakfasts and lunches. It worked out very well. Spending time in a romantic city with my husband was the best treat of all.

I've learned to replace the satisfaction I used to get from food with fun-filled moments. Keeping thin forces me to find other ways to enjoy my life.

I've also learned to cope better. In Santo Domingo, where the sugar cane grows wild, we experienced one disaster after another. We arrived exhausted at our hotel to find out that they were overbooked, and we were shipped off to a place on the other side of town. After changing our clothes, we looked forward to our dinner, which would give us a chance to settle down and relax. This was too much to ask. Our meal was abominable, to put it mildly. In the past, if this had happened, I would have eaten everything in sight to ease my frustration. But I didn't. Instead I told my husband how uncomfortable I felt, read a paragraph from a spiritual book, and we ended up laughing about the calamities of the day. What else could we do? We knew there was a better meal coming tomorrow and were sure we would find the restaurant that served it!

I have had to replace the enjoyment that food once brought me with other things.

If plans fell through, I learned to pamper myself by taking a warm bubble bath and calling a friend.

When alone, negative mind chatter would ultimately lead me to extra food. I gradually became aware of my destructive thought patterns:

- "I'm so lonely. Judy and Gale have dates tonight. There must be something wrong with me because I don't have one."

- "I have another ten pounds to lose, and it's coming off so slowly."

- "I want a better job so I can buy myself clothes, but nothing is on the horizon."

- "I'm scared because I feel so vulnerable lately—I don't know myself anymore."

Indulging in these thoughts were no-no's for me. If I caught my mind wandering, I knew that it would ultimately lead to my eating more food than I wanted to. So when these thoughts came up, I would tell myself they were dangerous and then call a friend or take a short walk to get out of myself.

What I've realized through the years is that I don't have to act on my feelings. I find strength in knowing that those "extra bites" ultimately will lead to misery and frustration. Gaining weight is not something I want to do.

I don't have to be ruled by my cravings anymore. I have friends to support me. And most importantly, I've developed an inner sense of well-being, which grounds me when all else fails. I can face life today without the food. If I were to choose between whether I wanted to experience my best day when I was overeating or my worst day now, there's no question in my mind that I'd choose the latter. Take a look; which would you choose?

	Best Day When Eating	Worst Day Now
Situation:	I was to have dinner with a colleague who happened to be a celebrity.	My husband's stepfather died, and the family was filled with grief.
What Happened:	All day at work, I obsessed about the evening's activities. Although it was a special event—being picked up in a limousine and dressing in my finest—I overate at dinner and felt nauseous for the rest of the evening.	I did not overeat and was able to help my relatives. (I packed my lunch and ate it after the funeral was over.)
The Result:	I was only half-present for the night, numbed out by a bloated feeling.	I was fully present and aided the family.

Taking the weight off and keeping it off is probably the most challenging thing I've ever done in my life. I was able to do it because I had support from other overeaters and could cope with every situation that came up. Replacing the emptiness I felt with love and understanding reassured me that *together* we would lose the weight and grow into the people we were meant to be.

Well, I've shared my heart and soul with you. If you relate to any of my story, you'll probably feel comforted in knowing that someone else has been there too, and understands.

I owe a great deal to the wisdom of the people I've met who are members of Overeaters Anonymous. Much of the material in this book comes from their sharing with me what has helped them stay away from overeating: namely, learning more about what their true needs are and how to meet them each day. I also cover the "tools" of the OA program in relation to how different members use them. I haven't gone into the 12 Steps of Recovery, which are essential to the healing process. If you want to learn about the 12 Steps, pick up some books that do discuss them.

Please keep in mind that this book is merely my understanding of how this wonderful fellowship works. I do not speak for Overeaters Anonymous. In this book, you'll also be privy to insights I've picked up along the way from many self-help groups to which I've belonged. Also, the food plans shared in this book are *not* meant for readers to follow. *Consult a doctor or nutritionist if you need a food regimen.*

1
It's Not Entirely Your Fault You're Overweight!

Our society is obsessed with being thin. We idolize the latest pop singer who looks like a rail. Our fashion models have prepubescent bodies. When we gain two pounds, we go into trauma. What price do we really pay for being crazed with weight loss and body image?

First of all, a lot of us are struck by body mania, and we are fat-obsessed. The National Center for Health Statistics reports that 34 million adult Americans were overweight between 1976 and 1980.[1] According to research studies, it's estimated that 5 to 10 percent of adolescent girls and young women suffer from anorexia and bulimia.[2] Even scrawny fourth-grade girls have complained that they weigh too much.[3] While we are dieting, our minds don't have much room to think of anything or anyone else. Dieters are usually preoccupied with how much they weigh or how much weight they have to lose. Do you recognize any of these "mind obsessors"?

- While sunbathing in the park, you think, "Everyone is looking at my fat body."

- At a fashionable party, while the waiter is coming around with treats, you think, "He can tell I'm the fattest one at the party."

- While hiking with a group of friends, you feel everyone is talking about how big your thighs look in Bermuda shorts.

- In anticipation of going out on a blind date, you think, "When he meets me, he won't ask me out again because I'm fat."

These scenarios go on and on, and I'm sure you could find another ten examples from your own experience. It isn't any fun to be fat-obsessed. We spend hours in wasted obsession. When I had this mind-set, I never really enjoyed my life. In fact, you might even say that when I was like this, I was going through the motions of life without really living.

The Diet's the Thing

What a rut we get ourselves into. We think that by finding the right diet, we will solve all our problems. How often have you said to yourself, "I need to find a diet that works, so I can take the weight off quickly"? But the truth about diets is that they never work over the long haul. As best-selling author Dr. Stuart Berger says, "Quick weight loss diets and gimmicks can get rid of excessive pounds, but the dieter is likely to regain this weight and the subsequent yo-yo gain and loss pattern compromises health."[4] Nevertheless, we take the weight off quickly, and we get frustrated when it comes right back on. Usually, we blame ourselves for not having enough willpower and become defeated. We cry out, *"Doesn't anyone have any answers?"*

As you'll see in the next few chapters, we overeat for a lot of reasons (and hunger isn't one of them!). But before you can explore those reasons and conquer your cravings, you must understand that it's not entirely your fault. Society has a way of messing us up. Mom says to clean our plates but tells us not to get fat or the boys won't like us. Women like men who eat the wonderful gourmet dinners they've prepared for them but prefer the lean, muscled look to a rounder form. Ads, TV programs, and movies show us nothing but ideal bodies, which are so depressing to watch that they're likely to turn even the most dedicated dieter into a refrigerator raider!

Furthermore, once you've been fat, it's hard not to get fat again. Dr. Jules Hirsch has done research on fat cells and the metabolic changes that take place within the body. When you lose weight, your fat cells don't disappear, they merely shrink. What actually happens is more complicated than that, but for our purposes, I want to emphasize that we always have the tendency to gain the weight back.

The problems we as a society have with fat and body image are well documented in books such as *Listen to the Hunger* and *Fat Is a Family Affair*. Feel free to pick up any of these books; you'll find them enlightening. But the main point to understand is that many things have led you to overeat. What you need now are tools to help you not to.

Later chapters will examine the dynamics of overeating and strategies to overcome personal food demons. But for right now, it is enough to realize that you have made a wonderful choice in reading this book. You have decided to stand up to all the conditioning that has "made" you overeat. Maybe you just got tired of being fat. Or maybe you are feeling especially low.

In Overeaters Anonymous, many members have described reaching this low ebb before entering the program. Take Florence, who was in OA for a while, left, and later returned:

"I had gone to a New Year's Eve party and was out of control. I was eating compulsively, doing cocaine, and drinking . . . . And I remember just lying in bed in physical pain—I just wanted to die . . . . I knew if I would come back to OA and reconnect with people, they would accept and love me right where I was. At that point, I was incapable of loving myself."

Or consider Henry, whose doctor gave him the final scare:

"The doctor said, 'If you don't lose weight, you're going to die.' I had high cholesterol and was a diabetic. I was frightened that if I didn't do something, I'd die."

You might say that Henry and Florence both were at the end of their ropes. In Overeaters Anonymous, many members share similar stories at meetings. Although some members may never experience the deep traumas of Henry and Florence, for many people hitting the bottom is realizing, once and for all, that they are sick and tired of being fat and are willing to do anything not to be.

'Fessing Up

Let me support you in facing the truth. Alone, it's too painful, but together we can do it.

Have you recently tried to lose weight but found you couldn't stick to your diet, even for a day? Do you find yourself feeling discouraged, thinking, "What good would it do to try this diet again?"

Are you willing to admit that, no matter what diet you try, nothing seems to work for the long haul?

Have you lost many of your friends because you don't

have the energy to give to the friendship?

Are you constantly depressed, unable to get out of this mood, finding it lingering for days?

Are you licked after taking a bite of something that you're not supposed to have?

Do you feel powerless when it comes to the food battle?

Do you feel resigned to live a life as a "fat person"? Do you tell yourself, "Fat is beautiful"?

Is there a "real you" inside who's imprisoned by your fat, just longing to come out?

If you've answered *yes* to three or more of these questions, you are probably feeling licked by your food problem. The admission of just how bad it is often is, ironically, the beginning of one's recovery.

A Little Bit of Willingness Goes a Long Way

All you need is a little bit of willingness to admit that the way you've been handling your food problem has not worked so far. It's scary to think that you are not as powerful as you thought. But you're *not.* Congratulations for being courageous enough to look at yourself squarely. Remember, you're not alone. Thousands of others have done it, too.

If you've made this admission, you're on the road to changing for the better. You'll begin to make better choices for yourself, but this will require a certain amount of honesty.

The path you are now embarking on will help you achieve the things you really want in your life. Many of us had been selling ourselves short, leading mediocre existences. We would go so far and no further. The pull backward was too strong.

To illustrate this point, let me tell you a story about myself. After losing all my weight, I bought myself a sexy new dress. But this 104-pound, petite body wanted her old tank dress back. It was more comfortable for me to wear than the new garment. However, there's good news to report. Sexy clothes eventually feel terrific to wear. You just need a little time to get used to them.

Despite the discomfort that often comes with growth, many OA members are committed to expanding their lives and reaching their full potential. To achieve this, they need a lot of help from their friends, as Natalie shares:

"My clothes fit no matter what season it is, but that's the least of it. I have wonderful friends, I date, I have fun times, and I travel."

And, on a more serious note:

"I really got more than I bargained for when I joined OA. There are words and goals in my vocabulary that weren't there before the program—words like compassion *and* acceptance.

"I pray every day to stretch my mind, heart, and soul. I'm trying very hard to be a little bit better, more flexible, more accepting of others and yet to strive for more discipline and to improve myself. I combine acceptance, discipline, and commitment. Commitment is not that ambitious drive for something, it's faith that sticking to a path will eventually produce a result."

So unlike what we've been told, reaching the bottom and feeling defeated is not the end of the world, but rather the start of a wonderful recovery process.

Join me in breaking new ground and becoming the person you are meant to be.

Notes

1. Van Itallie, Theodore B., "Health Implications of Overweight and Obesity in the United States," *Annals of Internal Medicine* 103 (6.2) 1985: 983–88.

2. Herzog, D. B. and P. M. Copeland, "Eating Disorders," *New England Journal of Medicine* 313 (August 1, 1985): 295–303.

3. Zaslow, Jeffrey, "Fourth-Grade Girls These Days Ponder Weighty Matters," *The Wall Street Journal*, February 11, 1988.

4. Berger, Stuart, "Doctor's Orders," *New York Post*, January 13, 1987.

2
When Food Calls Out to You

We all know what we should eat, so why don't we make the right choices?

If you're anything like me, you know what's healthy to eat: fish and vegetables have more nutritional value than a hamburger with french fries. We've been around long enough to read books like *Sugar Blues*, which deals with the harmful effects of sugar on the body, not to mention the psychological effects it has on some of us.[1] For a quick summary of this type of information, you may wish to consult the brief nutrition review in Appendix A.

Knowing what I should eat never helped me stop overeating. And all the scare tactics in the world—like, "If you keep gaining weight, you'll get a heart attack"—never kept me away from the food. I was powerless to stop on my own. Even though I had a lot of success in most aspects of my life, including my career, I was licked when it came to reaching for a cookie in the corporate cafeteria. Just one bite of something extra that was not on my food plan was enough to set me off. Yet, despite all evidence to the contrary, I still felt that I could control my problem by using a little willpower. But time and time again, I would try and fail.

I'd rely on a new diet to save me, but it couldn't sustain making the right food choices. What I know now that I didn't know then is that diets alone aren't enough to keep me away from overeating. I need lots of help from other people to keep my food problem in check. I know I'm not alone and that many people are like me. Maybe you're one of them.

Why Diets Don't Work

There's nothing more humiliating than buying a new dress, trying it on ten minutes before you're supposed to meet that special someone, and finding out that it's too tight because you've gained five pounds. "I've been so good on this diet; how did I gain the weight?" you say to yourself.

What dieter doesn't know this scenario? I sure do! The truth is that after all the struggle, deprivation, and frustration, you decided to take a few *nibbles* between meals—and these tiny morsels added up to unexpected mounds of fat. Instead of facing the situation squarely, you blame the diet—chanting every dieter's lament: "This diet doesn't work!"

How many times have you started a food regimen, lost control—started again, lost control—started again, lost control, and finally quit? A hundred times? Join the club. We've all participated in this broken record of failure, which leaves us depressed, believing that nothing will work. Nevertheless, when the latest diet doctor's menu appears in a magazine, we flock to the newsstands to buy it, hoping that *this* time we'll succeed!

I know your pain, because I've been there too. I wore my fat body like an isolation tank, dragging around two elephant thighs, which made me feel uncomfortable and self-conscious. The countless diet clubs I spent all my money on were for naught.

My pain wasn't in vain, because I'm here to explode the myth about dieting. Most diet books leave us disappointed because they make false promises and provide only a *physical reducer*, which isn't enough to sustain weight loss. Diets don't teach you how to love, express feelings of anger and jealousy, or help you to uncover your hidden fears. Instead, they usually lead to frustration because so many people can't stay on them for long periods of time, hence the yo-yo syndrome. It's a vicious cycle. And, if you're reading this book, you're most probably a compulsive overeater like me. I'm living proof that dieting alone won't make you skinny, self-assured, rich, and famous.

Most people who have taken weight off and kept it off (including me) have had to become aware of why they overeat and learn new habits so they don't go back to relying on excess food. This book is different from any other book you've read because we'll follow a group of courageous people through their daily bouts against the "tyranny of the bulge." We'll see how overeating is symptomatic of not being able to handle life's challenges. It isn't easy to learn to say *no* when you're used to saying *yes*. Or to risk losing friends by telling them how you *really* feel.

Compulsive Overeaters

It is possible to lose weight and maintain the loss. Many overeaters have done this. But making this happen takes a lot of self-awareness.

Most people in Overeaters Anonymous identify

themselves as compulsive overeaters. When they feel compelled to eat, they can't stop themselves from overeating. They are like alcoholics, who need to stay away from the first drink. As Dr. William D. Silkworth explains, "They cannot start drinking without developing the phenomenon of craving. This phenomenon, as we have suggested, may be the manifestation of an allergy which differentiates these people, and sets them apart as a distinct entity."[2]

I'm not a doctor, nor do I understand what happened to my body when I overate, but if I took that extra bite of something I wasn't supposed to have, as for an alcoholic, it would be the start of a lost weekend.

In a similar vein, Gilda, a vivacious lady, recounts:

> "I'd get up in the morning and be determined that today was the day I was starting my diet. I would start my breakfast with a piece of toast, a soft-boiled egg, and a piece of fruit. That was all I was going to eat. But I didn't stop there. Because I'm a compulsive overeater, just the taste of diet food triggered me off. I went from the diet food to—here we go again—to the box of cookies and other things. I couldn't stop. I kept eating all day long."

Milton, another OA member, defines a compulsive overeater this way: "A person who goes through periods where he binges on food, loses control, and may gain tremendous amounts of weight. Or he may purge himself and not gain weight. Food is an addictive substance, more than mere sustenance."

As Alice recalls:

> "I can remember being at the office, having been on a diet for a few weeks. I'd lost seven or eight pounds and was starting to look good. I was getting comments from people, and I felt good about it.
> "Then somebody would bring in a birthday cake. I would

tell myself, 'I'm doing really well on my diet, so I can have a piece of cake.' The minute I picked up a piece of cake, my whole focus was on food and away from life. I would start the binge, and it would go on for days, even weeks."

Many members talk about the fact that before they entered Overeaters Anonymous, when the impulse to eat struck, they had no defenses and would succumb to it. In the program, they may still crave extra food, but they have learned ways of coping with it.

As Alice explains:

"I remember standing in the middle of traffic, and the impulse to eat hit me, and I called my sponsor [OA buddy] because I just didn't think I'd make it. I said, 'I'm going to eat,' and she said, 'You don't have to.' I said, 'I do.' She said, 'All you have to do is to go home and get there safely and call me when you get back. I promise you, you don't have to eat.' She reassured me, and she led me the right way. I didn't hurt myself that day. Just a voice telling me that I could do it, that was all I needed."

Fred Schneider is an expert in the area of food addictions and eating disorders. I asked him why OA as a support group works for so many thousands of people. He stated:

Because they address the food problems and the necessary issues that have to change in order to do away with the symptom of those problems, the binge eating. OA doesn't address the specific problems; what it addresses is the need to change the way you deal with those problems. That is, you stop turning to food for the solution, and you start working on the problem itself.

Dr. Judi Hollis, Clinical Director of HOPE, Inc., a treatment center for eating disorders, refers many of her patients to Overeaters Anonymous. She writes that in OA,

> ... the sense of loneliness, uniqueness, and isolation is removed by regular attendance and forming a "home group." Hope is offered by others who have walked through the recovery process. A perspective is developed that despite immediate difficulties, things will work out. Depression is lifted. The program helps members maintain a positive attitude by first respecting and allowing feelings and then offering simple solutions as a program of ACTION. Fears are faced and walked through with group support. No one rests too long on their laurels of psychological insight with no behavior change.[3]

Part of the OA process is that members become more aware of their emotions. The meetings and telephone calls give them a safe place to share their feelings. As Stanley reflects:

> "Emotionally, I believe that with any disease of compulsion, when one picks up a binge item—which can be drugs, alcohol, gambling, sex, or food—at that age your emotional development is arrested.
>
> "I believe that anger is something one can binge on, too. I started binging on anger at five, six years old. When I came into the program, I was emotionally five years old, and if I didn't get my way, I'd throw a tantrum. The program has taught me 'easy does it.' No matter what happens, today is Monday, tomorrow's going to be Tuesday. Nothing is going to happen to me that's so terrible that tomorrow won't be Tuesday. And if something terrible does happen, I've learned how to deal with it."

Notes

1. Dufty, William, *Sugar Blues* (New York: Warner Books, 1976).

2. "The Doctor's Opinion," *Alcoholics Anonymous: The Story of How Many Men and Women Have Recovered from Alcoholism* (New York: A. A. World Services, Inc., 1976), xxviii.

3. Hollis, Judi, *To the Clinician* 1988. (*To the Clinician* is copyrighted material by Judi Hollis, Ph.D., and is available by calling 800-888 HOPE. No part or whole may be reproduced or excerpted for other works without providing attribution and ordering information as delineated by the author.)

3
Why We Overeat

Unfortunately, many of us have crossed over the line from eating to live—where food is sustenance that we enjoy—and we live to *eat*. Food has become all-encompassing, our greatest reward and our major defeat. We are obsessed with what we "shouldn't" have eaten or what we "should" eat for our next meal. Despite all this wasted worrying, we overeat anyway.

Fred Schneider, expert on eating disorders, has developed the following questionnaire.[1] Answer the questions and see if you share the problem of being food-obsessed. Answer the questions, and keep score as follows: never = 1 point, sometimes = 2 points, often = 3 points, always = 4 points.

Are You Food Addictive?

1. Do you get hungry when things are not going your way?

2. Do you find you get hungry when there doesn't seem to be anything to do?

3. After you have been frightened or scared about something that has happened, do you find yourself hungry?

4. When you feel "all alone," do you sometimes use food to get over the feeling?

5. After an argument with someone, do you find yourself wanting to eat?

6. Have you found yourself eating two breakfasts, lunches, or dinners because you felt the first was inadequate?

7. Do you find yourself planning the next meal before you have finished eating?

8. When you sit down to a meal, do you find you eat more than you wanted to?

9. Do you ever have a sense of being out of control during a meal?

10. Have you ever sought outside help to deal with your eating?

Scoring: Add points for each answer and compare totals. Below 15—you probably don't have a food problem. Between 15 and 24—food may be causing you some problems. Between 25 and 30—you seem to have a compulsive eating problem. Above 30—you may be a food addict.

If you're food addictive, don't panic. Throughout the

book, you'll uncover truths about yourself that may seem scary. But I'm not going to leave you high and dry; you'll also read about new coping mechanisms. *You are not alone*, so let's proceed.

What Secrets Are You Hiding?

Taking excess food is the last step of destructive action. There are many rationalizations we tell ourselves and uncomfortable feelings that surface, all leading to the overeating episode. To avoid compulsive eating, we have to take a look at what we have been hiding.

We all have things we feel we can't tell anyone about because we're too ashamed of them. About three years ago, I attended a workshop on empowerment, and we did an exercise where we sat in a circle and shared a deep, dark secret we had never told anyone before. The point of it was to let go of some of the ideas that keep us from enjoying our lives. Peeling off some of my isolationist skin felt terrific! It was amazing—none of the secrets were such hot stuff as to make the group cringe, and we all had experienced them at one time or another. So we're really not alone with our dark menaces.

It's time to face *your* moment of truth.

One of the most painful things about not being able to stop overeating is to think that no one else would understand. It's a self-imposed isolation, because we keep our deepest thoughts and feelings to ourselves. The pain of this type of existence is excruciating, and many of us know it well. If you identify with this attitude, know that you're not alone and that other overeaters have felt the same way.

Let's take a look of some of those "terrible" things you may be hiding:

- I hate my body and the rolls of fat I see in the mirror.

- I don't like myself very much lately.

- There's something that happened to me when I was a child that was so devastating that I can't forgive the people involved or myself.

- I sometimes feel suicidal.

- I blame other people for my own shortcomings.

- I feel like a glutton and get angry at myself when I overeat.

- I put on an acceptable front, but behind it all, I'm in a lot of pain.

- I have gotten into the habit of lying to myself and other people.

- I've done something recently that would hurt my family if they knew about it. The guilt is unbearable.

- I sometimes act as if I don't care about other people.

You make up your own.

Looking at yourself squarely, you see that losing weight involves more than a food plan. OA members look at compulsive overeating as a disease and take measures to treat themselves. This concept is a compassionate way of looking at the problem, because members don't view themselves as bad people but simply as people out of control when it comes to overeating.

However, when people are sick due to a physical ailment, a doctor can usually pinpoint the malady fairly easily. It's not so simple with the disease of compulsive overeating. It not only takes a toll on the body with the onslaught of excess weight, but it is also psychologically wearing, taking the form of negative mind talk. The "disease" may involve an assortment of destructive voices that are cunning, baffling, and powerful—playing havoc with our lives and asking us to deny what is really going on. Recognize any?

Voices of the Disease

"It's OK to overeat" (when you know you should not).

"You can have a little bit extra; it will take away the anxiety."

"Replenish yourself, feed yourself something sweet."

"You can go on a diet tomorrow— or anytime you want to."

"You're feeling great; you can let down your guard and celebrate with food."

"I make any depression feel better— just give in to me and eat extra food."

"I'm more powerful than your desire for health."

Discovering your own overeating patterns is one way of arming yourself against the "disease." It will make it easier for you to reach for health rather than give in to the disease. You'll have an opportunity to do this in Chapter 5.

Some of the Reasons We Overeat

Stress and Overeating

Our lives are often hectic—we have commitments to our family, friends, and career. How do we juggle it all? Often we pretend to know how to handle things when we don't, and, of course, we become stressed and burned out. Men and women today are breaking new ground. The old rules of dividing up responsibilities in the office and at home don't work anymore, and new ways of relating to each other need to be developed. This changing environment breeds stress if we are not fully aware of what is going on. In this condition, we are vulnerable to overeating, and food becomes a sedative for our anxiety. As you know, the added weight we put on only complicates matters and leads to greater problems.

Fear and Overeating

If we really face ourselves truthfully, one thing we all have in common is that we are afraid. All of us have our own personal assortment of fears, some of which have been with us from childhood. We may walk around unconscious of what they are, but you can bet that many of them surface daily—fears about never achieving our career goals, never meeting that special mate and having a family of our own. On a smaller scale, we feel anxious when asked to speak in front of a group because we feel that we don't have anything important to share. Or we feel inadequate, so we don't pick up a new hobby because we won't be able to do it as well as we would like. The list goes on and on—look at all the energy we invest in worrying.

The more we try to push our fears down instead of bringing them to the surface and exposing them for what they truly are—lies—the more food calls to us. How many times did I use excess food to give me the courage, only to find that it did nothing of the kind? I still had to face my fears, even with an extra ten pounds on my body.

Overeating as a Reward

Rewarding myself with food was something I learned to do when I was a kid. If I studied for an exam in high school, I'd take myself out for a Chinese dinner. If I made it through a horrible blind date, I'd come home to the cake in the refrigerator. If I had nothing to do on the weekend and worked hard all week, I'd stock up on my favorite ice cream, and on and on. My food would keep me company.

Let me state, now and forever, that I can't reward myself with food, because I don't know how to stop eating it! And these so-called treats ultimately led to my downfall. I had to learn other ways to pat myself on the back, which I'll share with you in later chapters.

In Chapter 5, when we examine your personal reasons for overeating, we'll explore other causes of this behavior. But first, it is important to realize that our food "triggers" don't have to run our lives. Many overeaters who realize the devastation that food has played in their lives have learned not to keep their realizations to themselves. Instead they get healing benefits by sharing them with a group.

OA meetings are like a safety net where people can talk about the things that they've always "eaten over." As Jane, a beautiful redhead, puts it, "I can come to a meeting and say anything. No one looks at me like I'm crazy." Al confesses, "I love food too much, and the only way I can stay away from it is to discuss my food obsession with other people." Here's what Alice recently shared at a meeting: "A few weeks ago, I had a major step in my growth process. I explained to my husband how angry I felt about what he had said. Years ago, I'd stew for weeks over the incident without opening my mouth."

Many OA members learn to live one day at a time. They can cope with anything that comes up in the day. They've experienced spiritual recovery, too. They have a faith in the goodness of life and have felt the presence of a positive force to help them with their destructive patterns of overeating. Whether it be the warmth of the group meetings or God, it doesn't matter. What matters is that it works.

It's hard to change channels, especially if you have convinced yourself for a long time that the right diet will work the miracle. But if you're anything like me, you've probably tried everything else—so what have you got to lose? Just some extra pounds.

Notes

1. Questionnaire excerpted from the book *The Food Addict* (unpublished manuscript) with permission of its author, Frederick S. Schneider, The Schneider Institute.

4
Hope and Glory:
Winners' Table

Gilda: Vitality and Chutzpah at Age Fifty-One

Gilda is one of the miracles in OA. She's truly inspiring—she weighed 256 pounds when she entered the program. She now weighs 128 pounds, and she's been maintaining this weight loss for thirteen years!

Meeting Gilda is a real treat. She's a powerhouse of energy and is filled with dreams and desires about what she wants to do with the rest of her life. Her aliveness, coupled with her phenomenal sense of humor, makes you feel uplifted when you're around her.

But she wasn't always this way. Before she entered OA, she felt as if life were passing her by. She says, "There was a thin person locked up inside of me, but I never thought she would come out." Her life was horrible and in many ways unmanageable:

"I'd have to go to fat-lady stores to buy my clothing. I couldn't walk up a small flight of steps without huffing and

puffing. I'd get terrible pains in my chest if I bent down to clean something. I couldn't fit into a bathing suit, and I was unable to get behind the wheel of a car.

"I come from a Jewish background, and my parents both ate normally. My mother was bone thin from the day I was born till the day she died. My father certainly could not have been called fat. He was an average individual.

"I'm an only child and come from a house where we were a little bit above middle class. My father was always in business. He had stationery/gift stores, and they all had candy in them, so my overeating started at an early age.

"My father had one establishment where there were fancy boxed candies—I remember Whitman's samplers in particular—you could see the flavors in the box. So you could start with your favorite and work down to something that really wasn't your favorite, but you ate it anyway!"

Gilda was a heavy adolescent, weighing 243 pounds at one point. Needless to say, her dieting career started at a very early age.

"I was on and off diets all my life, and when I reached age eleven, my father found a new doctor who lived in Jackson Heights, which was a long way from home. I was put on pills, which destroyed my appetite. That was good, but I also got a nervous condition, and my face would twitch from the amphetamines.

"I lost weight, and I looked normal—but not for long, maybe a couple of days. After I lost the weight, I thought I could eat anything and everything again.

"My father's next solution was to send me to a diet camp. He would grease the palm of the counselor and tell her to put me on a diet. I would lose thirty pounds away from my home environment, but as soon as I came back, I'd gain it all back.

"We tried everything—injections, diuretics. There was nothing my parents didn't try on me. In addition, my mother said to me, 'You know, nobody loves a fat girl, and no

one's going to want to marry you. You won't have dates with boys because you're too fat.'

"I started to get concerned about dating because I wasn't, and all my friends were. I was a very popular, outgoing person even though I was fat. I was very good with people, and I'd make them laugh, but none of the guys asked me out. I was always fixing up my friends with these adorable guys who thought I was very funny!

"When I was fifteen, we found 'Dr. Capsule.' (At that time, I weighed about 213.) He gave me the most beautiful capsules I'd ever had. They didn't make me twitch or shake. They made me very active, and they stopped the eating.

"This doctor was adorable. He made me feel that he really cared about me. It was easy to stick with it. I lost over 100 pounds. A whole new world opened up for me—I really was good-looking, and it was a totally different ball game.

"I met my future husband. We got married, and I wanted to have six children because I was an only child. During the pregnancy of my first child, I gained sixty pounds, and it was hard getting that weight off. It wasn't coming off, and I'd still go to Dr. Capsule from time to time. Whenever I took the capsules, I'd lose the weight, and whenever I stopped, I would eat.

"I had my second child two years later, and I gained sixty pounds that time too. After we had her, I said to my husband wait for the next one. We're still waiting for the third!"

Gilda was 256 pounds and a self-admitted "middle-aged Cinderella" with no life of her own when she reluctantly walked into an OA meeting.

"I didn't want to come into the program. A friend of my husband's, who had been an extremely obese person most of his life, ran into me at a party. He had joined OA three months earlier and asked me, 'How do I look?' I told him, 'Terrific.' He had lost fifty pounds in a month. He gave me

*his phone number and said, 'Please call,' but I never did. So
he called me and bugged me so much that I went to an OA
meeting—just to get him off my back!*

*"I listened to the things that people said, but I didn't
believe them, especially when they told me what they were
eating. Everybody was in the same boat, even though I
wouldn't admit it in those days. Everybody had the same
problem; everybody was a compulsive overeater. A compulsive overeater is a person who, when she starts eating,
cannot stop.*

*"Take me. I would get up in the morning and be deter-
mined that today was the day I was starting my diet. I would
start out with a 'diet' meal, but the idea of being deprived
drove me crazy. I ate and ate.*

*"Compulsive overeating is a disease, because it's some-
thing I did not ask for. I compare it to diabetes. People do not
ask for diabetes, it just happens to them. I didn't ask to be a
compulsive overeater, but if I had my druthers, I'll take
compulsive overeating over a lot of things out there, because
you can do something about it. For example, I would rather
be a compulsive overeater than someone who's blind."*

OA has taught Gilda new ways of coping with everyday problems.

*"It's taught me how to live one day at a time. I do not
worry about yesterday, because anything I did yesterday is
over and done with, and nothing I do will change that. So
why worry about it? I don't worry about tomorrow either. I
don't know if I'll be alive tomorrow, so why should I waste all
that energy? I try to live in the now. When I do, I'm free
from anxiety and depression. I can stand anything for one
day. I feel anybody can cope with anything for just one
day."*

Gilda's not the emotional type, but when she talks
about OA her eyes well up with tears.

"Overeaters Anonymous was much different than other weight loss programs I had gone to. People shared their guts and encouraged each other not to overeat, no matter what happened.

"For example, my younger daughter is engaged, and I had a very bad experience with my first daughter's engagement. She became anorexic for an entire year. Thank God for the OA meetings, where I could share the burden. I did not go back to the food, even though I felt tension, depression, and anxiety.

"My younger daughter has not become anorexic, but she has gone totally off the wall, completely crazy. She's an extremely sweet girl, but since she's gotten engaged, I don't know who she is. I started to worry. But I caught myself and said 'No, no. You went through this entire thing before, and everything is fine.' I refuse to let my younger daughter's ravings or whatever she's experiencing get to me. I need to keep her problems in their proper perspective, and I'm doing that right now on a daily basis."

Gilda's recovery in Overeaters Anonymous is a three-fold one: *physical, emotional,* and *spiritual.* As she puts it,

"First and foremost, it's physical. If you don't have the physical, you can't get the rest. Physical is the change from weighing 256 pounds to weighing 128. Your body changes, your appearance changes. You get happier. The thing that would upset me before the OA program was the fact that I didn't know whether I could refrain from overeating that day—I hoped I could diet, but I wasn't sure. That put me into a terrible depression. I don't have to worry about that anymore."

What did Gilda eat to lose the weight? Well, for one thing, she talks about a *Losing Food Plan,* rather than a diet. She sees a diet as a temporary thing, whereas a food plan is a way of life (more about this concept later on).*

> "My losing plan was four ounces of protein and one fresh fruit for breakfast. For lunch, another protein, a salad, and a cup of a cooked vegetable (or half a cup, depending upon the sugar content of the vegetable). Dinner was another four ounces of protein and a cup of vegetables. I would also have two cups of salad with two tablespoons of a dressing that listed sugar fifth on the label."

By the way, Gilda's maintenance food plan hasn't changed much.

> "I was a gourmet cook starting the program. On occasion, I still am for the family on holidays. But for myself, I keep it plain and simple. There's a saying in OA: KISS, for Keep It Simple, Stupid! When overeating is involved, I am, was, and could still be stupid. So I've learned not to fuss.
>
> "I also turned over my food for the day to a total stranger—told this lady I was working with, 'Tomorrow, I'm going to eat these three meals. I am not going to have anything in between them, and I'll have weighed and measured amounts.' I didn't have to worry about what I was eating; someone else was completely in charge."

As to the emotional and spiritual . . .

> "Emotionally, the program has helped. Abraham Lincoln said, 'You are only as happy as you make up your mind to be.' I understand now that nothing is as bad as it seems, so I 'turn over' my anxiety and depression. And that leads to the spiritual.
>
> "If you believe in God, that's good. OA is not a religious group but is a spiritual one. I came into the program a little

---

*The weight loss and maintenance food plans referred to in this book are only what has worked for some OA members. They are not meant for everyone. Overeaters Anonymous does not recommend or endorse any food plan. I suggest that if you are looking for a food regimen, you should consult your physician or a nutritionist.

bit spiritual, and I learned that when I wanted to eat something that was forbidden, to converse with a Power greater than myself (which I call God). I learned to talk to Him and say, 'Hey, listen, I have a chocolate cake in front of me, and I want to eat it. I was told by this very strange group, if I speak to You about it and ask You to lift this burden, You're gonna do it. Here's the cake I don't want to eat; don't let me eat it!"

"I don't know what came over me. I was able to take the cake and wash it down the drain. It works. I have learned to delay eating between meals. Even if I wanted an extra apple and it wasn't my time to eat, I would talk to God about it: 'Give me the strength to keep away from the apple,' and He did.

"Praying not only works with the physical, but it helps with every area of my life. You learn that things you go through in life—losing relatives, nasty people on the subway, your boss yelling at you, whatever—you can turn this all over and still come up smiling. I say to myself with any tragedy, 'This happened, but it's temporary. It doesn't have to happen forever.' "

Gilda has maintained her strength even during times of severe stress.

"After I had been in the program for three years, my mother died. I have no brothers and sisters, and my family is scattered all over the globe, none in close proximity. So here I was all alone.

"I found out that I wasn't alone. The word got around through the OA grapevine, and people came to visit me. I stuck to my food plan with the help of a Power greater than myself, who was truly taking care of me."

What are some of the things that Gilda does to stop herself from overeating?

"Something that has really helped me is taking an action when I feel the urge to eat coming on. When I begin to think *about foods I've never tasted because they came out after I joined the program, that's 'stinking thinking.' I have to take an action. I will scrub my kitchen walls and floors. I will get out of the house and run ten times around the block. I will start tap dancing up a storm. I'll go to an aerobics class. I take a physical action."*

Gilda also uses writing to clarify issues she's facing.

"Writing helps me clarify certain problems—I don't call them problems anymore, but when something comes up and you can't resolve it, then I guess it's a problem. But there is always a solution. In writing it down and thinking about it, I get it all out on paper. I get all my feelings up and out. If there are feelings of anger—anger is a biggie for me—I can put them down on paper. I feel so much better afterward."

Since Gilda has been thin for many years, it's important for her to remember what it was like when she overate so she doesn't repeat this destructive pattern. She keeps her memory green by working with newcomers to OA.

"I feel great when I give service to other people and it's accepted in the manner in which it's given. When people I'm working with 'get' the program, I feel as if it's happening to me all over again.

"I just got through to someone I've been trying to reach for many years. I ran into him recently and was shocked by his appearance. I had never seen him that size before, and I became frightened. He looked like someone who didn't have long to live. That obviously triggered something in me.

"I shared with him that overeating is a form of destruction. 'I was exactly like you not too many years ago, and I've found someplace that's created a completely different type of life for me. You don't have to do it alone.'"

On the homefront, it wasn't easy for Gilda to make Overeaters Anonymous a permanent part of her life.

"My family was not supportive of me in the program. I would pitch on this at OA meetings and tell members that my family didn't like the way I was eating or my spending time on the phone. I got strength in the OA meetings because I wasn't the only one facing this problem. Communicating with other people who were undergoing the same feelings made it easier. I learned early in the game that I have to be number one."

Milton: 150 Pounds Lost and Integrity Gained

Milton tells it like it is. He's one of the most brutally frank people I've ever met. But he wasn't always this way, especially when he weighed 450 pounds and was not in touch with his true identity.

"My earliest recollections of having problems with food go back to my childhood, around the age of ten. I'm Italian, and feasts were always occasions for celebration. I remember some of the most exciting times we had were when we used to go to both grandmothers' houses for Sunday dinner.

"We always ate well even though we didn't come from a very well-to-do family. You were healthy if you were robust and big. Being thin was viewed as being sickly. Food really did not become a major issue with respect to my weight until much later on in life. I wasn't an overweight child: I was very tall for my age. I was six feet tall when I was thirteen years old.

"I always used to look forward to the food; it was really great. At New Year's, my Uncle Joe used to make the most fabulous pizza in the world. I'd bring home eight pieces for breakfast. There was always a party atmosphere—the celebration was always around food. I was expected to appreciate—and finish—my food. I had to finish my meal before I could get dessert."

Athletics were always important to Milton, especially in high school, where he won many competitions.

"I was an athlete in high school and became very good at it, but was encouraged to eat a lot to develop muscles. This didn't make me fat; it merely bulked me up. By my senior year in high school, I weighed approximately 209 pounds. I was solid.

"My first experience with the scary side of food took place in college when I was about eighteen years old. I had gotten hurt and was unable to work out. As a result, I left school at the end of my freshman year at about 205 pounds. But when I came back at the end of the summer, I weighed 265 pounds! During those two months I had proceeded to hang out, drink, and eat a lot, and I gained over sixty pounds. Obviously, I had been getting away with not being physically fat because I had been an athlete and exercised all the time. So for all those people who overeat and keep their weight off by exercising, remember that it's going to catch up with you.

"I lost some weight and stayed at around 240 pounds for the rest of college. In 1963, when I got out of college, the draft board called me down. It was the time of the Vietnam War. They weighed me in at 255 pounds and classified me 1Y (overweight). I was given six months to lose weight so I could come back and be drafted. Of course, there was no way I was going to Vietnam. So when the doctor examined me six months later, I was 290 pounds. I was fortunate they did not take me.

"I stayed basically within the range of 270 to 290 pounds for about six years. I would reach 300 pounds and go to Weight Watchers and lose the weight very quickly."

Milton's professional credentials are very impressive, but developing his intellect never helped him control his food problem.

"I'm an administrator in a school for adolescents who are severely emotionally disturbed. My education is a master's degree, a bachelor's, and a professional diploma in administrative supervision. I'm currently going for a master's degree in social work.

"A number of things happened over the years. I got married, and it so happened that my wife was an active alcoholic. People often asked me, 'How come you didn't know she was an active alcoholic?' That's because we drank together, and I was drinking as much as she was. It's very hard to see the forest for the trees, especially when you're in the middle of the forest. I had very poor self-esteem. Because I didn't think I had anything to offer a woman, I married somebody I thought I could control.

"During this period, I tried almost everything to lose weight. I went to a diet doctor and got amphetamines, but I couldn't take them. I talk enough as it is, and with amphetamines, you couldn't shut me up. People would come into my classroom, and they never got out. They would be in there for two hours, and I'd be talking—they'd be trying to get out the door. I'd go on and on and on. I felt totally out of control with pills, so I stopped taking them.

"And I'd go and take some shots—I didn't even know what the hell it was—and I'd lose weight. I always lost weight when I 'dieted,' but I always gained it back, too. I wasn't able to sustain the weight loss. I'd lose weight when I felt lousy about myself, when it was beginning to threaten my self-esteem. There is a real close tie between how I feel about myself and what I weigh.

"I continued to gain weight while my wife was actively drinking. Our relationship was not good, especially our sex life. It wasn't her fault, it was our fault. We thought the solution to save the marriage would be to have a kid—out of the frying pan and into the fire. It did not do any of that. It actually made things worse.

"She began to get worse, and so did I. I would want her to get drunk so that I could put her to bed and I'd be free to eat. What happened is that my weight eventually went up to over 325 pounds. I met somebody while I was married, and we became lovers. She was probably one of the most signifi-

cant people I've ever known in my life. One of the things we did was to spend time together at night at Weight Watchers meetings.

"Weight Watchers played a major role in my life. I managed to lose weight. When I weighed in at Weight Watchers I was 338 pounds, and I went down to about 260 pounds. I would cheat, though, and it was a big joke, but I'd still lose weight. I got down to 238 pounds with their program.

"At that point my ladyfriend—who was married, by the way—had fallen in love with me, and it was mutual. There was just no way we could be together, though; there were too many problems. So her option was to move away and have a few children, a solution I had tried and that I knew didn't work. I was very angry at her, because this was the first person who had made me feel good about myself, made me feel sexual. After she left, my weight rose to over 400 pounds. By 1973, I had reached 450 pounds, and the reason I went back to Weight Watchers was that they were able to weigh me."

Then Milton found out about Overeaters Anonymous.

"A friend of mine who I work with invited me to a meeting. I said, 'Sure,' though I had no intention of going. I went home, and I ate that night. The next day I saw her and tried to avoid her all day. Finally, she said, 'I missed you last night. Where were you?' I said, 'I went home, felt tired, and went to sleep.' She kind of smiled and told me about another meeting on Thursday. I said, 'I'll think about it.' On Thursday night I guess there was nothing on television or I ran out of food. I was an hour and a half late, but I showed up.

"I walked into a room full of people. I was definitely the biggest person in the room. I stood behind the door in back of the room—trying to hide, which is difficult when you weigh 450 pounds. I wore a big coat, which covered my body, and

a huge beard concealed my face. I sat there, and tears came to my eyes.

"I think the thing that really touched me most was that I heard people say that overeating was a disease. It was treatable, and there was a solution. The solution was not simple, but there was hope. I didn't have to feel guilty about the fact that I had this problem, and a lot of other people had it too.

"Just knowing I wasn't alone was incredible. I was a very lonely man. My companions had been food and TV. I really had isolated myself from almost everybody at this point. I didn't go to any social affairs, I didn't see any of my family. I used to say it was because I didn't know if my wife would be drunk or sober. But that wasn't true, it was really me. I didn't want to bother with anybody. The more I ate, the more I isolated myself.

"I said, 'Wow, this is a great place to come and hang out—and it's free.' I really felt welcomed. I really thought, 'Gee whiz, these people like me.' That was a large part of the reason I kept coming back—they like me even though I thought they were all nuts. They liked me until I was able to like myself. They truly did offer me friendship, fellowship, acceptance, and they didn't care if I weighed 450 pounds. Janet, this very attractive older woman, came up to me, put her arms around me and hugged me as if she knew me. That was just wonderful, because nobody had done that to me in years."

Milton took the weight off with the help of OA members.

"An OA member said to me, 'Why don't you try to eat three meals a day and try to stay away from carbohydrates?' I said 'OK.' I would have an apple, a piece of cheese, or bacon and a couple of eggs for breakfast. For lunch I'd eat a few slices of American cheese, some bologna, a carrot, cucumber, tomato, and a cooked vegetable of some kind. And dinner would consist of the largest salad you'd ever seen in

your life, dressing, and anywhere from eight to sixteen ounces of protein. I would have a cooked vegetable sometimes, too.

"I lost weight—40 pounds my first month, 40 pounds in the second month, 40 pounds my third month. I lost 120 pounds in three months. In my first year in OA, I lost 200 pounds. Then my path was not straight and narrow, not perfect. Of the 240 pounds I lost in the first two years of program, I never put back 150 pounds of it. I've had problems from time to time, but I've really never left. Had I left at any point and walked away from the program, I probably would have put on that other 150 pounds plus. I've been in OA for fifteen years and have maintained a 150-pound weight loss for that time."

It's important to remember that compulsive overeating is a disease, and that losing weight is a process during which there may be setbacks. It isn't easy for Milton to maintain his wonderful body, especially when he doesn't get the attention that he did when he first lost the weight. Here's how he handles his maintainance. (Reminder: This is Milton's food plan. Each person needs to develop his or her *own* plan with the help of a doctor, nutritionist, or other qualified person.)

"I love yogurt, so for breakfast I have a cup and a half of it and a piece of fruit. Sometimes I change the yogurt to three ounces of hard cheese. I will, on occasion, have bacon and eggs—two eggs and two ounces of bacon.

"For lunch, I have a cup of salad, a cup of vegetables, a tablespoon of oil or butter, and six ounces of protein.

"For dinner, I eat six ounces of protein, a cup of vegetables, two cups of salad, and two tablespoons of salad dressing. Sometime during the day, I allow myself another fruit, which I may or may not eat in the course of the evening.

"Maintenance is a bitch, because technically you can eat more and maintain your weight. There's something very

strange about that. The issues are what do I want to add, what do I want to do? The worst part about maintaining is that nobody tells you how wonderful you look because you lost weight. It therefore forces you to look beyond the physical part of the program.

"I work with people who have carbohydrates at every meal or are macrobiotic, people who eat all kinds of things that I don't eat. I don't care what you eat. The issue is commitment, the letting go of your food obsession and not abusing food."

Milton has reached out to OA members to create miracles in his own life.

"I went to meetings. I spoke to people. I spent a lot of time with members in the program—that was the fellowship part of it—and I continue to do so. I went to two or three meetings a week. And my food plan gave me a direction, a guide to follow.

"People really offered me help. OA was not a business. I always questioned businesses. They wanted you to be successful, but the underlying motive was more financial than anything else, so I had some concerns about what they said. I didn't know whether I could believe them. In OA there is no profit motive. It's service, and service is given because that's how you keep what you got."

Milton also developed some attitudes that helped him get through the tough times.

"I felt that if I wasn't perfect, people wouldn't love me. I walked up to this fellow, Hal, who has been in OA about sixteen years, and shared how I felt after having a food slip. He said, 'So, it was one day. What are you going to do tomorrow?' I looked at him and said, 'What do you mean?' He said, 'Just because you had a problem today, don't throw away the last six months.' It wasn't great love or compassion, but it taught me a very important lesson—this program is *done a day at a time, and what I did yesterday doesn't count. What I do today counts.*

"To people who say they're eating and can't stop, I've said many times that you can stop if you want to. If someone calls crying, saying she or he has been eating all day, I ask, 'What are you doing now? You can stop right now. You're making a phone call—obviously you don't want to do it anymore. So what are you going to do next not to do it? Go to a meeting, make another phone call? Are you willing to make 20, 30 phone calls?' Some people over the years have been more willing to do those kinds of things. My path has been one of gradual physical, emotional, and spiritual growth."

Milton thinks of OA as a family.

"I've probably done more growing up in the OA meetings. In many cases, the people have been my mother, my father, my sisters and brothers—we've shared everything one might share. My blood family was always sabotaging me. I'm now remarried, and my new wife is very supportive— she's also in the program.

"What Overeaters Anonymous has done for me is to take my fantasies and turn them all into realities, and it continues to expand these realities beyond my greatest fantasy."

Bridget: No Visible Problem

Bridget was never very fat. In fact, you'd never guess she has a food problem. She's one of the many people who appear to be normal but are concealing a secret. As she tells it:

"I'm twenty-nine years old. I live with a roommate in New York City and work for a marketing firm as a manager. I grew up in a small, upper-middle-class town in Connecti-cut. It was a pretty homogeneous environment. I never

thought there was anything outside of this white, WASPy town. Actually, coming into OA I had to realize I was just like a lot of other people.

"I have six brothers and sisters and am in the middle, with three older and three younger. You don't have a lot to do, being the middle child. I went to the University of Connecticut and graduated with a degree in finance and was hoping to be a successful banker, but I found that marketing was more creative for me.

"I've gained and lost the same fifteen pounds every year. I was always sort of chubby as a child, but never fat. I used to be about five to ten pounds overweight as an adolescent. At college, about once a month I would binge on weekends. I used to call them mental health weekends. I'd take my groceries into the honors center, do my homework, and eat my binge foods. Then I'd go back to three weeks of regular eating.

"When I left college and moved out on my own, I would always have either good or bad days. The good days were Weight Watchers, Week One of weighed and measured meals. When I couldn't maintain that anymore, I'd go off, never eating really large quantities; it's just that I would make poor choices and would slowly gain about fifteen pounds. Usually this happened during the months of November to February. I'd then work very hard from February to April, when my birthday is, to lose the weight I had gained. I felt bad when I was eating anything that wasn't on Weight Watchers and good when I was able to keep on the diet.

"Last year, I joined Weight Watchers as usual in January, and I could not make a week. I'd try it for two days, then lose it and then join the next week, try it again for two days and lose it. It really scared me. My body was rebelling. That's when I came into Overeaters Anonymous. Weight Watchers didn't work for me anymore.

"I learned about nutrition in Weight Watchers, what

meals should consist of—three proteins, four breads, three fruits, and whatever. I also liked the group support. But I used to be a real Nazi with myself, and I would be very severe with my food because I wanted to lose the weight. If I wasn't losing, I wasn't satisfied. I would get bored with it—it was a diet, it wasn't a way of living for me.

"I started OA last year in January, so I have been maintaining the weight for about sixty days. I'm 5'5" tall and I weigh between 125 and 130 pounds, which is ideal for me. I used to weigh between 135 and 140 pounds.

"My food plan now consists of three moderate meals, and I pray to make loving choices about what I choose to eat. I know it's going to be like this for the rest of my life. I'm not concerned about losing weight today as much as I am about maintaining some level of consistency and having some sanity around my eating. A diet always was a four-week commitment to losing weight. It was like a course—having a beginning, a middle, and an end. I would just be able to stay on it long enough to lose the weight, and then I needed to jump off. It was always separate from my life. The food plan I have now is very much a part of my life; it's integrated.

"Breakfast is a cup of cereal with a cup of skim milk (I don't weigh and measure except for problem foods), half a cup of orange juice, an English muffin with butter. Lunch usually consists of a tuna fish sandwich with lettuce and tomato and a cup of soup. I have a snack in the afternoon of a banana and yogurt or just yogurt or fruit. For dinner I typically have half a chicken, a baked potato, a cup of vegetables, and a slice of bread. I eat a snack after dinner of yogurt and fruit or just fruit. It's amazing to me that I can eat what would be a heavy day on Weight Watchers—on Weight Watchers I wouldn't have the English muffin, baked potato, butter, a lot of things—but I can maintain a lower weight, eating the things I like.

"It's the consistency that's the key, knowing this is for the rest of my life. I don't feel as if I'm depriving myself at all. I don't deprive myself; if I want to have a bran muffin, I can if

I share that with an OA friend. If I want three cups of popcorn at the movies, it's OK too. (Popcorn I would measure because that could be a binge food for me.) I have pizza; I have everything I want to have. The blessing that I'm feeling now has to do with the fact that I can eat whatever I want and I'm maintaining. However, I don't eat sugar."

Bridget feels that abstinence—refraining from compulsive overeating—is a form of self-love. She has learned this new attitude by sharing with OA members.

"I feel as if I have a lot in common with people in OA, mostly due to my feelings of isolation, feelings of low self-esteem. I used to use food to fill me up, to keep me from feeling something I didn't want to feel. I relate very closely to people who share about that.

"Abstinence is making loving choices about the food I eat. I don't eat old food anymore. I used to eat old food because I didn't want to spend money on good food. I eat good food; I treat my body with respect. I feel I'm entitled to my three meals, and they are good meals.

"I don't know how this happened: I just walked into the OA rooms and learned to love myself and feel more entitled. When I used to binge, I would wake up in the morning beating myself, saying, 'You did it again, so today you're going to go on Weight Watchers and eat good food.' But by the time I got to the office, I'd already have had three doughnuts. Then I'd be on a sugar low and be lethargic. I really didn't give a damn about anything and was waiting for lunch.

"I was always able to maintain my weight because I would somehow get myself on a starvation diet and would lose five pounds . . . then gain back eight. It was back and forth all the time. Every time I put some negative food—some kind of carbo sugary thing—in my mouth, I'd physically feel the effects. Mentally, I'd feel awful for not having the guts or constitution to rise above that and have a salad. I was an extreme kind of person. My choices were either very *fattening, high-fat, high-sugar food, or something like string beans. There was no in-between.*

"People like me are in a lot of pain because we never let anybody know about our food problem. The people I tell I'm in OA say, 'Why? You're not fat.' So I have been very closeted about it. I always had to put on an acceptable front.

"Overeating never got in the way of my job, so I could rationalize that I didn't have a food disorder. Nevertheless, I would be struggling to keep my eyes open from the sugar."

Bridget talks about how she found out about OA.

"I was out to dinner with a friend who had been in the program for about two months. She started talking about the serenity that she had around eating three moderate meals. I saw her eat ravioli with a salad, and she talked about not being obsessed with the way she looked or the way she ate. That sounded like heaven to me. I decided I would go and see what it was all about.

"I went to an OA meeting and immediately judged everybody there. I said, 'Well, here I am. I've got a job, I'm successful, I don't have this problem. All these people are 400 pounds, or their hair is falling out, or they don't have jobs. I'm certainly not as bad off as they are, so why should I even come here?'

"I stayed away for a while, but my depression just got worse, and I couldn't control my eating anymore. I couldn't go on a diet. Instead of not being able to do a week of Weight Watchers, I couldn't even do one day of it, and that was weird.

"I went back to OA and saw a friend of mine from high school who I hadn't seen for ten years. She was sitting there, and I thought, 'Oh, my God, she sees me. I'd better run out of here. I can't let her know I'm coming to this meeting.' She was smiling at me, and I thought, 'You know, Bridget, either you're going to start to get honest about this, or there's no

place else to go.' And I decided then and there I was going to tell her about me and my food problem.

"She has turned out to be one of my greatest spiritual advisers, a really great support. I still felt the other people were a little bit crazy, but I couldn't deny that I was relating to what they said. I would go to the meetings and feel as if all I needed was a food plan that I could stick to, and I'd be fine. That was the great myth—that if I could just find the right food plan, then I'd be OK. I've been on every kind of diet ever created. What I've come to find out is that it's about getting honest and becoming a part of the human race.

"I lie about everything. I was a born liar. I lied about how hard it was to do a project, how much money I have—all to protect the image I want to put forth in the world. It's a very closeted existence. By coming out to my friend Betty, I realized that she and I were not so different. I had to acknowledge that I had the same disease she did."

Bridget describes what it feels like to be in the grips of the disease.

"It's a feeling that I don't belong in the world, and I should go hide under a rock or under the food. I identify with the people who say food is their friend. I used to spend my weekends going from deli to deli, just to buy the comfortable foods. If I didn't have a date, I'd sit with my pizza and Tab in front of the television, and that was my friend.

"In giving up my differences with other people, I realized I had to trust them. I had to trust that it was going to be OK for me to be myself. The feeling was like falling out of an airplane and hoping there was going to be a parachute. I often have the sensation of hanging on to the other members in the group when I reveal something. If I don't tell the truth, I'm going to return to self-hate and overeating. Saying something I detest about myself or revealing a secret, and having people look at me or smile, makes me think, 'Oh, my God, they accept me even with this!'

"One time, I had gone out to a benefit dinner in a Chinese restaurant. There were to be thirteen courses. I allowed myself to feel that this was too much to handle. The telephone has always been scary for me; 'Why would anybody want to talk to me? What do I have to say to them?' During the middle of my second course, I called a woman from an OA meeting, and I was on the phone with her for twenty minutes. She was so receptive. She had been somebody in a meeting who had said she needed to reach out more to people, so I felt it was safe to talk to her because I was helping her. I felt so much closer to her the next time I saw her, because we had been through a tough night together.

"Once I talked to her, it was fine. I didn't care what was on the table. I knew what I was going to eat, but somehow revealing it to someone else took the power away from the food. By revealing my vulnerable side, I got strength."

OA has helped Bridget with her emotional ups and downs.

"I used to get very depressed and spend weeks at a time thinking about how suicidal I was. (I was always so dramatic.) I would sit in my room and do nothing. The self-hate was so profound. To be able to feel the worthiness I feel today is something I had not anticipated I would get out of this program.

"Writing helps me stay positive. This morning I was feeling negative, so I started to write about it and saw some things had happened that I was using to beat myself up. Someone at work, a subordinate of a woman who wants me for this position, wrote me a nasty, caustic note that singled me out from everybody else. I couldn't stand the disappointment, and the truth is that she probably just had a bad day. I got up feeling as if I wanted to eat something that wouldn't have been a loving choice for me—like a bran muffin. Being able to stop and write about the incident made me select my *regular cereal, fruit, and English muffin. I was able to separate the feelings I had about the situation from my breakfast meal. I then stopped myself from throwing on my clothes and running out the door and said to myself, 'Why don't you do some more writing?' As I wrote, I also realized that my best friend was moving to Hartford, and she's thinking about having a family. I want a family! All these things came out in the writing.*

"By taking these few minutes, I was able to see my mind was full of these uncomfortable thoughts. I decided that I ought to take it easy that day because I was in a vulnerable state. I wouldn't have realized that if I hadn't taken the time to look at what was really going on."

The sense of belonging in OA was quite different from anything else Bridget had experienced.

"The intense loneliness I used to feel, the nights I was sitting by myself on the bed, staring at the TV with a Chinese dinner and feeling as if that was all there was to life—it was so painful. It's such a disease of isolation. I felt as if I was so different from everybody else, and I'm not. I affect other people, and they affect me. It's not about the food for me anymore.

"It's very humbling to realize I have this disorder. I know it's been lifted for these last two months, and it's been great. I thought being depressed was all that life was. OA helps me know I'm not alone."

These stories of some of the miracles in Overeaters Anonymous are inspirational. You can experience this recovery, too! A group such as OA provides the tools to support you in staying away from excess food and in reaching out to other people. You'll learn more about them in the chapters coming up.

5
Why Do You Overeat?

To obtain the insight necessary to move beyond food obsessions, you need to take a look at yourself in a new way. That takes guts!

Much of the information and quizzes you'll find in this chapter are eye-opening. If you're not used to facing yourself squarely, they may even seem confrontational. But the result of your answering these questions is that you will become more aware of what's involved in the vicious cycle of overeating.

Vacation Blues

If you find yourself denying your problems, the example of the vacationer will bring you back to reality. It is at these "fun" times that this destructive habit rears its ugly head, as any true "dieter" knows.

For me, vacations were often a setup for food trouble. It seemed OK to give myself permission to go off my diet, but the price I paid for it was too great.

Before and during a vacation, I would talk to myself with statements such as these:

- "I'm on a very strict diet because I want to lose ten pounds before my trip so that I can look great in a bathing suit."

- "How can I not eat those sumptuous meals on the cruise? I've paid for it, and I'm entitled to eat as much as I want."

- "I'll be very good at breakfast and lunch, which enables me to splurge on dinner."

Of course, after such a vacation I'd be sure to say, "I can't believe how much I ate. I gained five pounds on the trip. It wasn't worth it. Why did I do it?"

I think you get the picture. I had countless bouts with depression caused by vacation overeating. How many times have *you* acted out this scenario?

Food Obsession

Keeping the weight off is a serious matter. For me, that meant that my bulges became an all-consuming interest. From the moment I woke up, I was confronted with my oversized tummy. Then, throughout the day, I was thinking about what meals to eat and changing menus endlessly. How much time and energy do you spend thinking about your body, what to eat, and what not to eat?

How Much Time Do You Spend Thinking About Food?

---

1. Do you think about what you'll have for lunch just after you finish eating breakfast?

2. Do you constantly change your mind throughout the day about what you'll eat for dinner?

3. Do you find yourself thinking about food when you should be working?

4. Are your thoughts on something you'd like to eat when your close friend is sharing a problem with you?

5. Just before starting something new, do you look forward to what you're going to eat for your next meal?

6. Do you find it difficult to go shopping in a supermarket because you want almost everything in sight?

7. Do you get confused in restaurants about what to order for dinner and find yourself changing your mind more than once?

8. Are you finding it difficult to stop planning, thinking, and daydreaming about your meals?

9. When you're out on a date, are your thoughts on food, rather than what you're doing and who you're with?

10. Do you find yourself thinking about food when something enjoyable happens to you, like sharing a special moment with a loved one?

If you've answered *yes* to many of these questions, you're probably wasting precious hours thinking of food—not conscious of what is happening around you. Hasn't this food obsession taken a heavy toll on your life?

Overeating as a Substitute for Expressing Emotions

Most of my life, I had a plastic smile on my face—out of touch with what I was feeling. I smiled if someone was nasty to me, and I laughed when someone rejected me. Stated simply, I suffered from the nice-girl syndrome.

I ate to cover up my feelings of anger, fear, sadness, and loneliness. Today I'm in touch with my emotions. I know when I'm angry and have learned to express it— even if it comes out awkwardly. I love, cry, and feel afraid a lot of the time. This marvelous mix of sentiments is what, in part, makes up *me*. Years ago, as an overweight person, I became what I thought others wanted me to be. Now I am a transformed woman—and you can be, too.

It's important for you to become more aware of your feelings and learn new ways of expressing them. Discovering your emotional self may be uncomfortable at first, especially when you've been used to eating to hide your feelings. Who among us can experience anger, fear, loneliness, and sadness when we have been busily trying to please other people? Most of us never learned to take care of ourselves and get our needs met. When we become more aware of what we need, it may seem overwhelming.

What has helped me during these times is to know that there are other people who share the same feelings and don't know how to deal with them. It's also comforting to observe that, over the last sixteen years, I've never experienced anything that I couldn't handle with the help of other people.

Fear

At the root of our feelings is usually fear—fear that we will lose something we already have, or fear that something we want is unattainable. Isn't this true? Recall three things that you were recently afraid of. Don't they fall within one of these categories?

A few years back, during a self-realization seminar, the leader asked twenty-five of us to come on stage and remain silent. Not one word was uttered, yet our minds were going a mile a minute. Each of us had a different scenario ticking away. Underneath all this thinking was utter terror. We were petrified of each other. Without our so-called personalities to hide behind, who were we? Fear is part of the human condition, not particular to any one person. Take solace in the fact that you're not alone.

Myth: If you do "it" the right way, there will be no fear.

That's a lie. Fear will always be there—in intimacy with friends, trying something new, asserting yourself— whatever! By allowing for it in everyday life, you diffuse its power to paralyze you. And by sharing your fears with other people, you won't have to "eat" them down.

Felicia, an attractive executive in her late thirties, was terrified that she might not succeed at her new job.

"In the middle of the day, I would be paralyzed with fear. I was supposed to be making phone calls, and I would be sitting there pushing papers around because I was panicked. I would pick up the phone and say to an OA friend, 'I'm totally panicked. Everybody else is working, and I'm sitting here pushing the same piece of paper around.'

"It helped just to have somebody sitting there on the other end of the line, saying, 'Oh yes, I know exactly what you're talking about,' and to hear somebody laugh and then suggest, 'Do one thing—tell me one thing you're going to do!'

"I'd tell that friend an action I was going to take and then hang up the phone. Strangely enough, I was productive for the rest of the afternoon."

One way of coping with a fear attack is to verbalize what you're afraid of to another person, as Natalie does.

"I think verbalizing it helps immediately, so I'll talk to somebody about the guy I'm going out with and how afraid I am to date him. It makes me feel that I'm not isolated or alone, that there's someone else who has gone through the same issue, or maybe is going through it now."

▶ ▶ ▶ **HELPFUL HINT** ◀ ◀ ◀

Imagine your fear taking the shape of a furry animal. Speak to it, and tell it that it can't take you over.

Anger

If we added up 100,000 pounds of human fat and looked for its psychological cause, we'd find it to be anger—anger at our boss, family, the checkout clerk at the supermarket, or whoever else (you fill it in!). What do we do with this feeling? We stuff it down with food.

Anger almost never strikes alone. It's usually accompanied by feelings of rejection, hurt, loss, or fear. Recall the last time you were angry. Wasn't that the case? The following examples will help clarify the dynamics involved.

Situation	**Feeling Behind the Anger**
I'm furious when my husband takes me for granted.	I feel *hurt* and *rejected* when he doesn't treat me the way he did when we first met.
My sister always gets the first choice of everything. It makes me so angry!	My family doesn't really care about me. I feel so *hurt*.
My boss takes out his frustrations on me, and I'm furious about it.	He reminds me of my father. Nothing I do is ever good enough. I feel so *frustrated* by this.

My two closest friends are going out together, and they didn't invite me along. I feel like giving them a piece of my mind.

I feel so *rejected* when they don't include me in their plans.

I'm so furious at the way my date treated me. I don't deserve to be talked to that way.

Why am I so *afraid* of standing up for myself?

▶ ▶ ▶ **HELPFUL HINT** ◀ ◀ ◀

When anger strikes, take a look behind it.
Try to identify what other emotions you're
feeling. Share the insight with a friend. Your
anger may dissipate.

Sadness

Many of us run from feeling sad—either by suppressing it with food or by numbing it with constant activity. When we stop overeating, a lot of sadness may begin to surface, because we mourn the lost years caused by burying our "real" selves under layers of fat. We need to be very gentle with ourselves at this time. Dwelling on wasted time doesn't help much. A more compassionate way of dealing with the past is to realize that food was our only recourse at that time; we coped with situations the best way we could.

I've learned to embrace the part of me that grieves as if it were my child. I actually imagine a sad " 'Lene," crying and feeling very frustrated. She's about eight years old, and she wants to be loved. I then picture Helene, the woman, nurturing this little girl and saying to her, "I understand how you feel, 'Lene. I'll take care of you." Helene wipes the tears from 'Lene's eyes, and they hug each other. (I might do this exercise ten times a day if the need arises, and it usually does.)

▶ ▶ ▶ **HELPFUL HINT** ◀ ◀ ◀
The next time you feel sad, begin to
nurture all parts of you. Give *your* "child" a
name, and talk to him or her lovingly.

Loneliness

Growing without using excess food to numb the pain is
a lonely process. We find ourselves needing to take
leaps of faith on many occasions—not knowing where
we are going to land. We attempt to handle the unknown, bumbling our way from one situation to another.
Yet we pick ourselves up and proceed anyway, discovering new "muscles" we've never used before. We
begin to listen to that small voice within us (our intui-
tion) and follow its guidance. We don't need a hundred
people to tell us what to do anymore. We have the
answers.

If we change the word *loneliness* to *aloneness*, the mean-
ing shifts. Loneliness means that in some way we are
not complete in ourselves, not enough. Aloneness im-
plies that we can stand on our own as a whole and
complete person.

How do we create this change in perception in our
lives? It starts with awareness. The following examples
will help to clarify the difference.

Loneliness	Aloneness
I hate being by myself on a Saturday night.	I have myself and the things I love to do. My time alone can be quite fulfilling.
I feel so lonely in the midst of the party.	I don't feel connected to the people here, so I'll make an effort to reach out to one person.
I ache from not being with a "special someone."	No one can fill the emptiness in me. I need to fill it with love for myself.

Now that you have some ideas about how to recognize and respond to your emotions, let's take a closer look at your feelings and frustrations.

What Has Overeating Been Covering Up for You?

Which of the following statements apply to you?

1. I'm angry at my boss (co-worker) but can't tell him or her about it, so I reach for food.

2. I feel so overwhelmed by life at times, and I reach for food.

3. I'm lonely and frustrated on Saturday nights, so I reach for food.

4. My aunt (or any other relative who acts as a host or hostess) gets upset when I say *no* to the main course, so I reach for the food.

5. My mate (lover, parent) doesn't understand what I need from him or her, so I reach for food.

6. When I feel sexual, I get scared and reach for food.

7. I'm in debt, spending money that I don't have, so I reach for food.

8. I've just moved in with my lover, and our lives revolve around his or her schedule, so I reach for food.

9. I'm getting older and haven't yet accomplished my career (social life) goals, so I reach for food.

10. I don't have time to sit down and eat normal meals, so I reach for food.

11. I've just graduated from college (or reached another turning point) and don't know what I want to do in life, so I reach for food.

12. I have to take care of the family and have no time for myself, so I reach for food.

13. I find it difficult to say *no* when I want to and end up doing things reluctantly, so I reach for food.

14. I'm drained and feel spent, so I fill myself up with food.

15. There are so many uncomfortable feelings coming up, so I deaden the pain with food.

Unmasking the Lies
By understanding my feelings better, I uncovered certain lies I told myself. Many of them seemed contradictory. In one moment, I could be certain about something that made no sense ten minutes later.

Untruths That Led Me to Overeat	What I Found Out to Be True
No one understands me.	I never gave people a chance.
No one has problems as terrible as mine.	I was so self-centered that I wasn't aware of what people were going through.
I'll never achieve my dreams. I feel so alone. I might as well overeat.	There are so many people that feel as lonely as I do.
My problems don't count.	I count as much as anyone else.
My life is meaningless, so I can't help myself when it comes to overeating.	I've learned so much. It feels terrific to be able to help others.

My life has no real purpose.	No matter what happens to me, my life is about helping other people. I have received a lot, and I need to reciprocate.
The only real pleasure I get comes from eating my favorite foods.	Having friends and building a relationship with my husband feels so much better than food ever tasted.
I can't trust anyone.	No one is perfect, but others can be there for me some of the time.
I feel such shame and guilt because I can't control my eating.	I have a disease called compulsive overeating, and I need to take special care of myself.

When I began to understand my true feelings, I was able to realize that I was distorting reality and began to recognize the truth. If you will be honest with yourself, the same thing can happen to you.

Loving Myself Back to Health

I cringe when I think of all the aggravation, mortification, and basic frustration that the extra weight on my body has caused me. What I lacked—especially when I overate—was self-respect. If I became fatter than I wanted to be, I condemned myself mercilessly. What I desperately needed was to have compassion for an imperfect me, no matter what my weight was.

6
Putting Recovery First

You may be thinking, "The word *recovery* in the chapter title is too extreme to apply to me. I only have a small food problem," or, "I don't have that much weight to lose."

Even if that's the case, aren't you hurting too? Chapter 2 showed how devastating overeating can be for many people. Take a good look at your own life. Are you as fulfilled as you'd like to be? Haven't you been using food to hide certain feelings you've been afraid to acknowledge? When we are overeating, we're really only half-alive!

According to *Webster's Dictionary*, to recover means "to bring back to a normal position or condition." How many of us have used food normally? Not me! So recovery *is* an appropriate word to use.

A more important question to ask yourself is, "How do I get myself back to a sane eating pattern?" Unlike a diet program, Overeaters Anonymous offers a threefold recovery process:

1. *Physical recovery*—the weight comes off!

2. *Emotional recovery*—not "eating down" feelings

3. *Spiritual recovery*—feeding the inner hunger appropriately

First Things First: Physical Recovery

Recovery starts with staying away from excess food. As Felicia says, "The first thing is to be a healthy, normal weight, whatever that is for you." When I was close to 160 pounds, I had no respect for myself. My over-stretched, gluttonous body wasn't exactly what you'd call dainty. The more I hated what I looked like, the more I overate. I didn't see any way out of the depression I was in.

When I was at my heaviest, I wouldn't buy any new clothes for myself. I rationalized that if I did, it would mean that I'd be staying at this heavy weight indefi-nitely—my life was on hold! I'd wear my old reliables, whether they fit the occasion or not. Since they were all that I had, they became like uniforms—holy relics, in constant use!

What I had to learn was to love and respect myself at any weight—even 160 pounds! This was no easy task and took a lot of coaching from friends. I even broke down and bought myself an outfit at 150 pounds. That in itself was miraculous.

I also practiced talking myself into "right thinking." For example, I'd look at my face in the mirror and say, "You look terrific today" (whether I meant it or not). I remember a friend of mine saying, "Just don't eat, no matter what happens to you." Her caring got me through many a sleepless—potentially, snacking—night.

If you are on a safe program, the excess weight will come off exactly when it is supposed to. Fat is like a protective skin—as you are ready to cope in a new way with life, it sheds itself.

Staying on a Food Plan

The key to staying on a food plan is loving yourself enough to do it. You can start at any time, even if you've recently gained weight. Know that you are a worthy human being—regardless of what the scale says. When the "I weigh too much blues" hit, treat yourself lovingly, perhaps using the following examples.

Situation	Alternative to Eating
You've gotten on the scale and see that you've gained three pounds. You're so obsessed by this occurrence that you can't concentrate on anything else.	Instead of falling apart, you call a friend, who tells you, "You're not what you weigh. See what happens next week when you get on the scale."
You're at a party and glance at yourself in the hall mirror. You've gained so much weight that you feel like a pig. All you can think about is going home.	After you see yourself in the mirror, you think, "I'm not where I want to be, but I will get there. I'll go over to someone and strike up a conversation."
You're at a family barbecue. It's the first time they've seen you in months, and you're at your heaviest weight. As a result, you feel like eating everything on the table.	Self-respect at any weight means loving yourself regardless of how others react to you. To arm yourself for family affairs, bring a supportive friend along.

Choosing a Food Plan

A food plan is an important element of a weight loss program. Unlike a "diet," which you go on and off, a food plan is a sane way of eating that can be modified to fit your lifestyle when you reach your goal. Learning to eat with sanity involves discipline. You practice eating three meals a day, and each meal has a beginning, middle, and end. In contrast, when I was overeating, I would eat just one "meal"—which would go on all day.

There is no one food plan that works for everyone. In Overeaters Anonymous, members are on a variety of regimens—whatever works for each person. This book won't offer you a food plan either. As I have suggested before, you should contact your physician or a nutritionist for advice about what to eat. What I can give you is the encouragement that you can succeed, despite the discouragement that you may feel because of past failures.

To help you get started on a food regimen that's right for you, it's useful to look at some common misconceptions about what guidelines we think we should follow. See if any of the following misconceptions sound like choices you have made or been tempted to make.

Food Plan Misconceptions

The Truth

"None of these food plans seem right to me. I have to wait until I find one suited to my needs before I start my weight loss regimen."

Waiting to find the "perfect" food plan will only get you fatter. It's best to pick a sensible plan and get down to business. You can always modify your plan as you go along.

"I love to eat _____ (fill in the blank), and this food plan *includes* them, so I'll try it."

It's dangerous to love any food too much. If you're looking for a regimen that contains all your food turn-ons, you're only fooling yourself about losing weight. Look for a sensible plan that doesn't include your binge foods.

"I won't be able to stay on this regimen. It will take me months to lose the weight. I want to find something that will let me reduce quickly. This won't do it."

Deprivation "diets" can create fierce cravings for the foods you miss. You could end up gorging on them and gaining back more than you took off.

"I feel so constricted on a weight loss food plan because I don't have my 'treats'! I realize how much I use certain foods to fill up the empty spaces in my life."

By putting food in its proper perspective—a source of nutrition—you will be able to meet your needs for companionship, love, and excitement with friends, hobbies, and other appropriate outlets. Ironically, sticking to a food plan can give you a lot of *freedom*. You won't find yourself ruled by the fear of overeating anymore. No matter what you feel at any given moment, it has nothing to do with what you put in your mouth.

"I know I can stay on a food plan at home, but how am I going to manage my food at a business luncheon? People will laugh at me when I don't eat and drink what everyone else does."

By sticking to what you are supposed to eat at business luncheons, and paying attention to the conversation, you'll find that people aren't really interested in what you are eating!

You can see that most excuses are unproductive. So don't delay. Just select a food plan and get started. Understand that there is no such thing as perfection. Looking for the perfect food plan only postpones getting on with your life and losing weight. Remember, nothing is etched in stone—if a regimen isn't right, you can change it later on.

A food plan should be flexible and suitable for all occasions. This is very important if you want to stay committed to your food regimen. Don't pick something that is so rigid that you have to be a monk in Tibet to stay on it!

A food plan requires discipline. The discipline required by a food plan is that we follow it. But contrary to what many of us think, it doesn't have to be constricting. In fact, it is *freeing*. By knowing what you're supposed to eat and eating it, you have more energy to devote to the wonderful things life offers you, like being with friends and enjoying yourself.

A food plan should not include your binge foods. If you don't want to set yourself up for failure, avoid foods that "turn you on." If you binge on sweets, don't select a food plan that allows you to have desserts. You may even want to set limits on foods that you've had problems with in the past, like cheese or cereal. Weighing and measuring these items can prove helpful.

Your commitment to a food plan is just for *one* day. This is the key to success. It's easier to stay on your food plan if you think you'll do it for *one* day. Tomorrow will take care of itself. Your goal somehow becomes manageable when you break up time into small chunks. Also, be sure to take all the actions that will help you not overeat *today*!

Remember that a food plan alone won't make you thin. It is only one element of your recovery.

Emotional Recovery

The last chapter talked in great detail about the range of feelings that come up when you stop covering them over with food. It takes courage and time to face our emotions and deal with life in a new way. For some people, therapy proves very useful in dealing with this.

Spiritual Recovery

When you stop overeating compulsively, a void is left. Many people experience this as a sense of low self-esteem, loneliness, or a profound "inner hunger," which may come from a lack of nurturance in your earlier years. A lot of love and compassion from other overeaters, friends, and therapists can heal these old wounds. For many OAers, the group is their first introduction to a concept called "Higher Power," an alternative voice that counters their destructive tendencies to overeat. It becomes a force that helps them choose health rather than the disease.

For many, a belief in a Higher Power goes beyond the group—some people choose to call it God, other people describe it as a cosmic force. It's a highly personal concept—one person's belief may be totally different from another's. While OA is not a religious group, most members come to believe in a form of spiritual recovery. Let's take a look at what some OAers recount about this experience.

Henry, a nonbeliever turned spiritual, says,

> "I ask God to put an angel before that first bite and me. And if I want to give up and quit today, He helps me not to overeat. He's never failed me.
>
> "I want to get closer to God. I want to be a channel of love, become less fearful. I'm not concerned about accomplishing success or making a lot of money. I want sanity and to serve people—to lose my self-centeredness and my self-will. I want to contribute in life. That's success."

Natalie's worrying about dieting stopped when her concept of God changed.

> "Whenever I'm in serious trouble or any kind of deep problem, the way I keep from eating is to pray, and it always helps.
>
> "Even as a very little girl I believed in God, but for some reason I thought God would punish me because I was bad. With all the problems I had, I didn't know what I did wrong and became very angry at God for not explaining.

"I read Rabbi Kushner's book When Bad Things Happen to Good People, and that was a real spiritual awakening for me. From that point on, I didn't overeat anymore.

"Rabbi Kushner's son died at the age of fourteen of a very rare disease. He, as a rabbi, had to question God and his Jewish teachings. If somebody dies, you rationalize to a child that God needed that person more than you do. But kids as well as grown-ups tend to doubt this and to wonder whether they did something wrong.

"What I got out of the book was that I didn't necessarily have to believe that God would punish me for doing bad things. That was only an idea, and there are many ideas about God. Kushner's idea about God was that God is All-Loving. I immediately abandoned my old philosophy and took on that new one—a real turning point for me. For six months, I didn't worry about dieting. I didn't worry about any kind of weight loss at all. I just concerned myself with eating healthy foods."

Stanley, an ex-atheist, recalls,

"I would ask myself, 'Why don't you believe in God?' I'd answer, 'Because I'm an atheist.' I have a scientific background, and if I can't weigh and measure something, it doesn't exist.

"I was having a conversation in my head, which I remember as if it were yesterday. I said, 'OK, then what would it hurt if I listened to the other side?' For the first time I listened, and I thought, 'Just maybe these people have got something.'

"At that exact moment, I can't explain it, I can't even describe it, but God came into my life. Just by my saying that maybe He exists. It's as if I opened up the door a crack, and He came rushing in. It was a spiritual experience for me. It was not something that later on I turned around and said, 'Yeah, that must have been God.' It was something that I felt right at that moment."

Sandy (a Wall Street executive who joined OA to lose weight and found unexpected benefits):

> *"I'm not superstitious but I believe that there are no coincidences, and I'm here as an example of what this program can do. Everyone knows you get thin by eating less. And I wanted to get thin, that's why I came into OA. But I believe you can have a serene food plan and experience peace in your life. That's the real appeal. Today, I feel in close contact with God."*

As you might have guessed, recovery from compulsive overeating is a full-time job and requires a lot of work. But the rewards are many—a new body, self-respect, and a confidence that comes from truly loving yourself.

7
Abstinence

Weight loss involves discipline. I can't drive home this point enough! Meals don't go on forever. They have a definite beginning, middle, and end. And they don't contain everything you want to eat. (We've all tried that, and it doesn't work.) It's useful to space your meals three to four hours apart as well as to plan for them. Plan, don't get obsessed. There is a difference!

Planning vs. Obsessing

Planning means shopping for a variety of foods so you can make your meals easily, as well as arranging to share some of them with family and friends. This is much different from changing your mind three different times about what you want to eat for dinner or who will accompany you. This type of behavior can be obsessive.

You've probably been on all sorts of diets where you felt deprived. And the day you lost your weight, you ate everything in sight. A food plan (as opposed to a diet) is a way of eating for the long term, and it may change according to your needs. For example, as you lose weight, you may want to take back some of the foods you had not been eating. But there's continuity in using a food plan. As Stanley puts it,

> "A diet is something you're going to lose weight on. It's a form of deprivation so that you will be able to get down to that perfect weight and be that perfect person, and then you'll be able to eat all those fattening foods to reward yourself. When you're on a diet, it's a kind of self-flagellation.
>
> "A food plan, on the other hand, is a way of stroking yourself. It's something enjoyable that you never have to go off of. There are some foods I'll never eat, because I know that they're not good for me. I don't eat candy or red meat."

Some OAers find that they need structure, while others seek flexibility. Again, there are no formalized food plans that Overeaters Anonymous endorses.

Many OAers whose relationship with food has been particularly chaotic find that they need structure, definition, and discipline in their food plans. Yet they also require a certain amount of flexibility to fit in comfortably with their lifestyles. Other overeaters come from extreme rigidity and control and benefit from introducing more flexibility into their eating regimen. Here are some examples of both types of people.

> "I've tried to eat moderately, but I don't have any success. I start out OK, but my food gets sloppy. I need more structure with my food."

> "I come from a very rigid place with food. I need someone to listen to me talk about my food but not tell me what to eat. My food plan has a lot of flexibility. I don't commit to exactly what I'm going to eat at each meal, but I share generally

what I'll have—for example, protein, vegetable, and salad for lunch."

"I feel much more secure writing down exactly what I'm going to eat each day. This way I can't fool around with my meals. I need a lot of structure. Without it, I get confused, and that leads to overeating."

If you are unclear about what you need, keep observing your behavior around food. Share your insights with other overeaters. Through this process, you'll begin to know what is right for you.

To simplify matters, write down what you are going to eat that day. It's an antidote for "food fogginess" and keeps decision making simple at mealtimes.

When in doubt, leave it out! That means simply that, when you're unsure of something that you might want to eat, don't eat it. We sometimes become so confused about our food choices—to the point of obsession— that we forget what Scarlett O'Hara's simple solution might have been: "There will be another meal *tomorrow*." But, in all seriousness, if we're trying to reclaim a view that food is just a source of nutrition, what does it matter if we don't have a certain something today? With this philosophy, we can experience *life* between our meals. Isn't that what we really want to do anyway?

Keep Your Memory Fresh

Very often, the more distance we put between our destructive overeating patterns and a sane way of eating, the more we tend to forget how "bad" it used to be. We really never have this thing licked anyway. So, I keep a picture in my mind of what it was like the last time I overate. I don't have to remind you of what this unpleasant picture was like—you must have plenty of your own memories.

Abstinence for the Compulsive Overeater

Abstinence is one of the key tools that many compulsive overeaters use to refrain from overeating. As we discussed earlier, a compulsive overeater needs to stay away from excess food the way an alcoholic can't pick up a drink. Alcoholics can have a hard time overcoming their disease, but at least they can finally come to the realization that they can't drink *at all*. They put a cork in the bottle, and they don't have to deal with liquor anymore. With overeating, it's more complicated. We all have to eat to stay alive!

In terms of eating, abstinence means different things to different people. Here are some common definitions of food abstinence:

- Making loving choices about food
- Eating three weighed and measured meals a day without eating anything in between
- Staying away from the first compulsive bite
- Refraining from compulsive overeating
- Guilt-free eating
- Binge-free eating
- An organized, disciplined way of eating
- Three moderate meals a day with nothing in between
- Sane eating
- Having a food plan you've committed to someone
- Following a plan of eating that is healthy and sane
- Taking only one helping during meals
- For hypoglycemics: eating five small meals a day

- Sticking to a food plan
- A way of eating that's not whimsical and that nourishes the body

Ultimately, you must decide for yourself what abstinence is. Although overeaters may guide each other and share what has worked for them, they don't have the answers for anyone else.

The process of learning about what's abstinence for you is not an easy task, and every overeater needs to find his or her own way. But the journey is exhilarating, and in Overeaters Anonymous, men and women can share their experiences and compare notes.

"Less" Is More

Despite the seeming contradiction, when you cut back your excessive eating, you'll receive *more* in the form of feeling better about yourself. And you'll lose weight too! I used to "brainwash" myself to believe this, and after a while, I actually did lose weight. It proved to be true!

Sandy describes the process of how she created a sane way of eating, which not only helped her lose weight but enabled her to enjoy meals.

"I targeted a food plan and asked myself, 'What would make me comfortable? What would make me eat this way for life? Forget the diet, the weight, and the numbers. What would make me not panic at the thought of doing this three times a day for the rest of my life?' And that's how I evolved my food plan, with bagels and an occasional sandwich and a glass of wine.

"Once a month, I got on the scale to see where I was, and when I got down to around 125 pounds, I looked pretty good. Then I coasted for a while. I reached a new degree of willingness a few months later. It wasn't an upsetting thing.

No one ever raised the issue; just all of a sudden I would say, 'Sandy, you're ready to cut back a little.' That idea brought my weight down to 115."

"I made a list of things I was entirely ready to give up, foods I might be willing to give up, and items I'd never be able to give up. Every week, I would pick one or two and eliminate them from what I was eating. I'd leave myself the option at the end of the week to renege and say, 'Forget it.'

"Some of these items were very small. For example, I might decide, 'I'm not going to eat the olives in my Greek salad.' Since I was eliminating one or two foods every week, my efforts accumulated, and I lost weight. I was eating a smaller fruit, a tablespoon less of dressing, so very gradually—without feeling deprived—I took off more weight, finally reaching 115."

▶ ▶ ▶ HELPFUL HINT ◀ ◀ ◀

Here's an opportunity for you to do what
Sandy did. What are the items you're willing
to give up, might be willing to forgo, and
never will be ready to do without?

Willing to Do Without	May Be Willing to Do Without	Never Will Be Willing to Do Without
1. _____	_____	_____
2. _____	_____	_____
3. _____	_____	_____
4. _____	_____	_____
5. _____	_____	_____

Willing to Do Without	May Be Willing to Do Without	Never Will Be Willing to Do Without
6. _____	_____	_____
7. _____	_____	_____
8. _____	_____	_____
9. _____	_____	_____
10. _____	_____	_____

Not all members become abstinent right away. It can take years, as it did for Natalie. Some members are luckier, and it grabs hold quickly. Ruth knew her way of eating was "death," and she was ready to do *anything* that was suggested to her.

The many payoffs of being abstinent are summed up by Felicia:

"I gained absolute freedom to enjoy my life and my work, to enjoy the people I come in contact with, because I'm not thinking about food all the time. Some days I look at my meals, and nothing seems enough. But for the most part, I look forward to my life. I don't have to worry 'Did I eat too much or too little?' I eat comfortably, and when the meal is done—it's done!"

8
Sharing

Whether it be with Overeaters Anonymous, another support group, or just a gathering of your friends, *sharing* with others and letting them know your secrets can take the edge off old isolationist patterns. In realizing that you don't have to be perfect and that other people are available to help an imperfect you, you start the process of *breaking down*, which will ultimately allow you to *break through*.

Needing Other People vs. Isolating Yourself

I remember reading a story called "Go Away Dog" to a kindergarten class. The tale went like this:

A little boy has problems in dealing with other children and his family. People get angry at him, and he's left alone a lot. He finds a stray dog on the street and tells it to go away. Yet the dog insists on following him around. At the end of the story, the boy makes a final plea to the dog to go away. But just after he says that, he tells the dog that he loves it and wants it to stay.

The little boy was me in a nutshell. Most of my life, I put up barriers between myself and other people, never acknowledging how much I cared about them or how much they cared about me. Food was a convenient buffer. It didn't talk back, and if I felt hurt or rejected about something, I could "eat it away."

Many of us are this little boy to some degree. If we stop our running (through overeating) and summon up the courage to take a look, we find that we need other people. Love was what I really needed, and food was a poor substitute for it (no matter how delicious it was). I longed for a sense of connectedness to other people. I had always felt like an outsider, the "black sheep" of the family. And I created this scenario in the office and with friendships. Overeating fueled my negativity.

How often I'd be alone—stuffing down my feelings with food. The loneliness was sometimes excruciating. I thought my situation was so terrible that no one could understand it. How wrong I was. I didn't realize then what I know now. I'm not unique. Many people feel the way I did.

Next time you go to a party, take a good look at the people who seem so together. Look beyond their image of success and self-sufficiency. We're all in the same boat; we need caring and love from other people. We lose sight of this when we reach for food, alcohol, or drugs to fill an inner emptiness.

Florence, for example, remembers the loneliness of her adolescence.

"There was never enough food to fill that void, the hole I had. The hole would say, 'You're not enough. You're not good enough.' It was low self-esteem.

"I remember being left out by friends. Everyone would go out and play or call for each other, and I was never included. I would try to force or manipulate my way into being with

people. When I was rejected or not included, I would go home and eat. It was a very lonely, isolating experience. I was blocked from other people; there was no connection at all."

Natalie, a successful businesswoman in her late thirties, explains how she used food to cut off her feelings.

"Food is really the only way I know of cutting feelings off from myself. The last twelve years have been a process of learning how not to do that, undoing all those nasty habits of covering up my feelings with food.

"If you could experience the worst physical pain you ever remembered, including breaking a leg or having a tooth trauma, multiply that by a hundred—it doesn't even come close to touching the emotional pain of overeating. I'd start thinking about my meals and what I was going to eat, and on and on.

"I obsessed over my job, people, places, and things, too. Either I was in the past, regretting it, or I was fearing the unknown."

Many overeaters have isolated themselves with food instead of experiencing the fullness of life. When they enter OA, they realize what they've been missing. As Alvin suggests:

"In the course of two years in the program, I've learned there's a different kind of death, the death of the soul, life, and spirit. I now see that refraining from overeating is living life and not blotting it out. I see life as filled with pain, conflict, and worry, but I can take the steps to be abstinent through it all. And I don't have to do it by myself. By being clean, I get to experience the joy as well as the pain—the absence of things that can hurt a lot. I'm in touch with reality. When you overeat, you are not only denying the painful moments, but the pleasurable ones as well."

By giving up compulsive eating and getting more involved in the mainstream of life, you become less self-absorbed. Life becomes more meaningful because you share a common bond with others and have a sense of being needed. But with any gain, a loss is involved. In this case, you lose the excitement of what it's like to live on the edge.

Many overeaters describe themselves as having addictive personalities—wanting everything or nothing, having little patience with themselves or others, and always living at extremes. But once they are on the recovery path, things seem to get calmer and more serene. They experience the healing power of *love*. This powerful force allows them to discover their true selves, straighten out their family relationships, and have more fulfilling friendships—a tall order, which takes a lot of time.

For most people, the sense of isolation is broken when they come into Overeaters Anonymous. They don't have to go through anything alone anymore. This usually involves a process of learning new things about themselves. Alice, an attractive young woman who looked as if she had it all together, first had to learn what her interests were at age thirty-five.

> *"I didn't know any other activities besides overeating, so I didn't know how to have new expressions of myself. I had to try what other people told me they did for recreation, to see if I liked it.*
>
> *"I started opening up more, sharing more, going to movies, doing things that didn't revolve around food. That took the focus off the food. It was hard for me to get started. I didn't know how to begin."*

Old Wounds Die Hard

Not only do overeaters need to look at themselves and become more aware of what they want, but they also need to understand how their destructive behavior has hurt their family and friends. With the support of other people, overeaters can work through this painful realization and learn to develop new guidelines for dealing with others.

For example, one woman shared how she used to get a lot of attention from her family when she overate. Everyone was concerned about how unmanageable her life was. She no longer enjoys playing the victim, and when she goes home, she tries to be more a part of things. Also, as Milton said earlier, he no longer needs to retreat into overeating when involved with an intimate partner and is learning to deal head on with the problems that come up. The process of healing yourself and restoring relationships or creating new, healthy ones takes time and requires patience. The support of the OA group is invaluable and teaches overeaters self-love.

Breaking Through in Overeaters Anonymous

OA meetings are an opportunity for members to practice self-acceptance. When a group of overeaters congregates, humility and truth surface. Often hearing other people speak about the feelings you've been hiding from yourself allows you to take a look at yourself.

Meetings are alive and vital—a safe place for members to share their feelings. Many people have not worked through adolescent problems because, when they were younger, they used food to stuff down their feelings. Now, they have an opportunity to work through those problems. Meetings are a haven from the outside world. For many, Overeaters Anonymous serves as a bridge back to life, helping people to cope with their feelings so they function better in everyday life.

A lot of soul sharing goes on—a true nurturing. Once you get a taste of this, you want more and more of it.

Henry, one of the old-timers, describes the healing energy in OA meetings. He encourages people who are still struggling and have never experienced OA.

> *"Get into the meetings quick. Sit . . . soak . . . you don't have do anything. Just soak. Keep coming back. Just give yourself a break—a chance. You've got to get better, and it does get better."*

If you were to walk into an OA meeting, you'd probably see in the span of the hour and a half someone crying, lots of gut sharing, people laughing, and many members hugging. You'd feel an electricity in the room—a warmth—that can't be put into words. A special something that you'd want more of. Let's experience part of one of these sessions:

> *Scott, a handsome man in his late thirties, shares how difficult it is for him to reduce the amount of food he eats. He wants the reward of having a thin body but is reluctant to let go of more food. He has already lost ten pounds but refuses to take away any more "little extras."*
>
> *Joan, a young woman in her late thirties, begins to speak. Her voice is shaky, and tears are streaming down her face. In a low voice, she confides to the group that her father recently died: "It hurts so much. How can I get through this time without overeating?" She asks the group for support: "I could use phone calls from people."*
>
> *Neil, a successful fifty-year-old executive, talks about how difficult it is for him to keep to his food plan when he's out of town on business. He recently returned from Kentucky and is glad to come back to his "home group."*

Sandy, the young Wall Street executive we met earlier, makes time for meetings wherever she goes.

> *"I go to about three a week. I've gone to meetings in Tokyo and London. I get a sense of consistency and belonging by going. It helps me to see familiar faces year after*

year. It keeps me in touch with the fellowship, which I find enormously supportive."

Natalie talks about how, by going to meetings, she overcomes a sense of isolation. She'll even cancel a business appointment to go to a meeting if her abstinence is threatened. After all, she won't be fully there for her clients if she's overeating. In talking with other overeaters, she is there for *herself.*

"I go to meetings several times a week. They make me feel that I'm a part of a larger plan. People understand what I'm going through, and it keeps me from feeling isolated. When something severe happens to me, such as my parents being sick, I go every day, no matter what.

"When I'm under stress, I change my entire lifestyle and go to more meetings. If I don't secure myself in the fellowship, I'll go back to overeating. I've been abstinent going on four years now, and it took me eight and a half to get there, so I don't take it lightly. To make sure I don't creep back into old habits, I go to a meeting every day.

"My abstinence comes before anything else. I cancel a whole day of business if I think I'm going to overeat. I don't get immediate relief from one meeting. It's a collection of constantly going that makes me feel a part of OA and God's greater plan. Going to meetings and sharing about what I'm going through is a great relief."

Felicia feels that the meetings are a safety net for her.

"I totally belong. At meetings I get in touch with the real me—the me that wants to be happy. When I feel that I want to overeat, I go to a meeting, and the desire to do the number is just lifted out of me."

Anonymity

Not only can you share what's on your mind, but no one will tell anyone about it. That's right, overeaters commit to following a tradition of the program called anonymity: "What you see and hear here, let it stay here!"

Moreover, anonymity means that everyone is on a first-name basis. At beginners' meetings, this tradition is explained further: "If you see someone from OA walking down the street with another person, you don't acknowledge that he's in the program, but just say 'hello.' "

In this way, people can feel secure in talking about whatever or whomever they want to, without it getting back to their friends and family. There's a camaraderie among members, a caring, a sense of fellowship, a feeling that they are all part of a team. Together they can lick their food problem and life's challenges. It's amazing that a food disorder can be a catalyst for this feeling of usefulness and team spirit.

Types of Meetings
There are all sorts of OA meetings. Here are just some of the different types:

- Beginners' meetings—to introduce the program to beginners

- Abstinence workshops—dealing with the challenge of abstinence

- Step meetings—based on the 12 Steps of Recovery

- Big Book meetings—based on Alcoholics Anonymous literature

- Discussion meetings—addressing themes of everyday life

▶ ▶ ▶ HELPFUL HINTS ◀ ◀ ◀

Do at least one of the following:

- Go to an OA meeting soon. If you have a problem

with overeating, or another type of eating disorder, you'll be welcome.

- Start your own meeting. All you need to begin are two other people.

- Join some other type of support group.

Phone Calls

"Reach out and touch someone." Isn't that what phone calls are all about? In OA, many members rely on the phone. They use it as a "mini-meeting" between meetings. Most members start a phone book of group members and collect numbers so that they can call people for support at all times of the day and night.

The phone becomes like a lifeline and has helped many OAers reach for support rather than food. It's wonderful to know that someone on the other end of the phone will reassure you that a piece of cake won't make your boss speak to you with more respect and that the only thing a pizza will do is make you sure that whatever you really want *won't happen.*

Many OA members find that their phone bills increase once they enter the program. But they feel that this is a small price to pay for the recovery that they have received.

Sophia talks about how she was terrified of calling people early on in her program. Her sponsor suggested that she make at least one phone call a day as a way of learning to reach out to others for help. She would call and simply ask the other person how he or she was doing. The conversation would then turn to her, and she began to let others know how she felt. Now you can't keep her quiet; she shares at every meeting!

Really sharing yourself with other people is harder than you may think. Many people find it easy to make polite conversation, but to let someone know how you really feel is another matter. The telephone is a useful tool that with practice can offer you the opportunity to tell the truth.

Stanley was skeptical of making phone calls at first. He didn't understand how it would help him stop overeating. But now he's a true convert—it helps him stop overeating all the time.

> "I've built a support network, people I know are there for me. I try to surround myself with the 'winners.' That's not grandiose or egotistical. I want powerful, productive, positive people in my life.
>
> "Anybody I call will tell me, 'You know, I get hungry too, but I don't have to eat. You don't either.' It doesn't matter what we talk about—the football game or how insidious this disease is. We might even talk about my mother's combat boots. But after a little while, the obsession to overeat lifts. I don't know why; I haven't got the foggiest clue."

Alvin relies on the phone, too.

> "I always make calls. Being in contact with others helps me all the time. One of the things that amazes me is that if I'm helping somebody else who's in trouble, or able to give them some insight, I feel terrific having done so. Somebody I talked to this morning was very angry at himself for having spoken harshly to his young daughter. He apologized at the time but still felt lousy. I simply said to him, 'You're not perfect. None of us are perfect. You did let her know that you felt sorry, that you didn't mean to hurt her.' After we spoke, he was able to be a little easier with himself. By my giving to him, I really gave to myself. I figure, if I'm telling him to be easy on himself, maybe I should do the same."

Florence has gotten through many traumatic experiences by using the phone.

> "Just last week my grandmother and uncle died within two days of each other. I made a phone call to someone and said, 'I can't deal with food. Please plan my food.' And this

person told me what I was going to eat for breakfast, lunch, and dinner. The onus of making decisions was off myself. People were really there. I got so much love—lots of phone calls."

▶ ▶ ▶ HELPFUL HINTS ◀ ◀ ◀

Try these telephone tips:

- The phone is a lifeline. Start viewing it that way, and call someone when the urge to overeat strikes.

- Make at least one phone call this week to someone you don't know very well. For starters, say hello.

- Call a special friend when you're bothered about something. Let it all hang out.

- If someone calls you needing help and you don't want to be bothered, take a minute out to talk anyway.

- Share something wonderful with a friend this week. Call him or her unexpectedly.

9
Sponsorship

In the last chapter, we discussed sharing and the breaking of old behavior patterns. In this chapter, we are going to deal with a particular type of relationship that has helped many an overeater put the food down. This person is called a *sponsor*.

Help Is on the Way

Did you ever have a best friend to whom you could tell your darkest secrets? A buddy—someone who was on your side? Maybe it was a parent or a mate. This person supported you in being yourself. You didn't have to pretend with him or her.

That's what sponsorship may become. A sponsor is usually someone who has been around longer than the newcomer and can guide him or her through the OA program. Even old-timers have sponsors; they are an invaluable source of support. You may have more than one sponsor: one to talk about your food with, a work

103

buddy, a person to help you with relationship issues, and one to guide you through the 12 Steps of Recovery.

A sponsor is empathetic and understands the mixed emotions that arise when one stops misusing food. And there's no question of status in OA—a corporate vice president may be sponsored by a secretary.

A sponsor usually gives the sponsored person "tough love"—"tell it like it is" feedback. Natalie explains this concept further.

> "I get fired by more people than you can imagine. I really don't take nonsense, and what I offer is what I've done. I essentially say, 'Are you willing to do what I've done?' Initially, they say, yes, but when we go about attempting it, I get a lot of flak.
>
> "I sponsored somebody who used to tell me what she was going to eat each day. She had difficulty sticking to what she said, so we agreed that if she couldn't turn over specifics, she would give me general food groups and amounts. But she still couldn't do it. When I asked her why she changed her mind, she said, 'I felt like it.' She eventually told me that she didn't want to call me anymore. A year later, we spoke, and she apologized.
>
> "It was important for me to stick to something I committed myself to. As a compulsive person, I would flit from one thing to another—one food to another—gaining and losing weight constantly. Keeping to my commitment gave me an organized, disciplined way of handling my food. When you learn how to keep your food in order, you learn how to keep a lot of other things in order, like your feelings."

Sandy talks about the value of being sponsored and sponsoring.

> "I speak to a woman who has been abstinent for about twelve years. We speak at the end of the workday, seven days a week. She calls me around five o'clock. If one of us is out of town, we try to stay in touch, but we have to wing it

sometimes. . . . We have a conversation for about five minutes. If other issues need to be discussed, we may take a little extra time or make a plan to talk later. For example, I'll say, as I did today, 'I have a business breakfast at the Continental Hotel. They're usually pretty good at bringing me fruit and cottage cheese. Yet I always have to be prepared for the unexpected! Once they showed up with a Danish, coffee, and juice. In the worst case, I don't have to eat breakfast. I also have a luncheon meeting at the Gloucester House.'

"She said, 'Oh, good, that's a fish place.' I told her I didn't have school tonight and expected to have a regular dinner at home.

"She encourages me to be flexible, and I resist that, so the daily contact is helpful in trying to turn this stubborn person around. The repetitive nature of a daily contact will break down any addict's resistance.

"I weigh myself once a week, and when my weight goes up, I panic. We've created a rule—you're not allowed to change your food plan on the day you weigh yourself. You have to stick to what you've committed to. This helps me, especially when I'm waddling and want to eat air for breakfast and cancel my dinner plans. My sponsor encourages me to accept my weight fluctuations.

"I've been sponsoring for eight and a half years, my entire time in the program. I believe that it's an important service, giving back what you've been given. I try to establish long-term relationships with those I sponsor. It's funny; over the years, my sponsor has also become the person I sponsor. We take turns—a little Jekyll and Hyde.

"I sponsor three people. The helpful part of being sponsored is that you can share the mass confusion, guilt, and anxiety of the last twenty-four hours. For example, one woman can't handle going to salad bars. Yet she goes anyway! I have a historical memory of her food and remind her of this pattern. I'm in a position of trust with her, so I maintain a certain formality in our relationship."

Letting Go

As you have seen, with a sponsor you can turn over what you're going to eat that day. It's a relief knowing that someone else has heard your commitment, and you don't have to worry about food—you've already decided what to have. And for the skeptics, there's something about listening to another compulsive overeater speak from the heart—it's irresistible. You begin to trust him or her, and that makes life a lot easier. No one's perfect, but OAers try hard to be there for one another.

Sponsorship is about letting go of control—not having to do it all, know it all, or be it all. It feels uncomfortable at first to give up a behavior pattern that has helped you survive, but in time, it becomes wonderful knowing that someone else is there. Atlas can finally release the weight of the world from his hands and join the human race!

▶ ▶ ▶ HELPFUL HINTS ◀ ◀ ◀

To establish your own sponsorship, follow these steps:

1. Call someone who can serve as your sponsor for one week.
2. Commit to calling him or her at least once a day. Set up a time when you will speak.
3. Tell him or her what you're going to eat that day. (Write it down beforehand.)
4. Share with him or her any particular food problem you might anticipate (going to a certain restaurant, being with a family member who's always pushing food on you, and so on).
5. Try to be open to your sponsor's feedback. (It will probably help.)

6. Be honest. Share what is really bothering you. You get out of things as much as you're willing to put into them.

7. Don't be afraid to let your sponsor know anything else that's on your mind—for example, "My boss asked me to work late tonight, and I'm angry!" Nothing is too trivial—these are the things that have led us to eat compulsively.

10
To Life!

When I was in my twenties and "eating down" my feelings with food, life seemed hopeless. How could it be anything but, when my greatest enjoyment came from what I fed myself? Overeating ruled my life, but eating sanely over the last sixteen years has unleashed a new me filled with vitality and excitement. I now look forward to the surprises of each day. One of the greatest gifts I have received throughout the years is to experience love, which is a powerfully healing emotion.

Many of us run from this intimate feeling, even though it is the thing we want the most. Sal, a recovering overeater, shared such a reaction with me.

"I was always running from myself. I just hid in the food I ate. With some recovery, I got more sophisticated, and I used my anger to separate me from other people. It allowed me to keep a 'safe' distance.

"But when I looked beneath my anger, I discovered that I was using it to cover up a mass of fear. Much to my

amazement, I was terrified of almost everybody and every-
thing. In desperation, I was forced to press beyond the fear. I
found that beneath it was a lot of love. So this 'terrible
monster' I thought was me turned out to be a teddy bear."

Like Sal, when I'm the neediest—needing "strokes"
and hugs from other people—I often retreat into my
anger. In the past, I used to get something from it—
"negative attention." But more and more, I realize how
unfulfilling this is and am learning how to ask for what I
really need—caring from friends.

Learning to Love Myself

Practicing new behavior isn't easy, and I have had to act
as if I knew what I was doing every step of the way. My
friends guided me and were there when I reached out
to them. Here are some of the suggestions they made
on how I could take better care of myself:

● When I was too hard on myself for making a
   mistake, they said, "Take it in stride, give yourself
   credit for risking. Next time you'll know how to
   handle a similar situation better."

● They told me to do something nice for myself at
   least once a day—something that would make
   'Lene (my inner child) happy, such as buying myself
   a small gift, taking myself to the zoo, something
   frivolous just for me!

● They told me to become more aware of the
   negative messages I tell myself and substitute
   them with positive thoughts. For example, I learned
   to replace "You're fat—you'll never lose the
   weight!" with "You're doing a great job sticking to
   your food plan."

● They encouraged me to take a look at the things I

did for myself each day—*not* the things I didn't do, which only made me feel worse.

- They suggested that I look at my wardrobe, throw out old clothes that were worn, and replace them with new and lovely things.

- They supported me in developing friendships that could nurture me: "Just go for coffee with one new person this week."

- They taught me to rest for a few minutes during the day when I felt stressed. For most people, taking care of their bodies in this way was routine. But I had to learn how to take time out for myself.

- Although I needed to become aware of my anger and find new ways to express it, they pointed out to me that I'd feel more serene if I could detach myself from the person, place, or thing I was mad at. Holding onto resentments was dangerous. I wasn't a terrible person because someone didn't treat me right. Maybe he or she had a bad day, so why should I take it personally? (This is easier said than done.)

- They taught me that my opinions are important and that I have a lot to contribute in my professional and personal life.

Identifying Imbalances

As I loved myself more and more, I began to shift my priorities. I realized that I would have to create a balanced life for myself if I wanted to reach my full potential. Reevaluating my priorities became most important. I had to look at how to divide my energy and time between developing my career, sharing myself with family and friends, and exploring new hobbies and interests. I noticed that there was an imbalance in my life because I had been putting too much emphasis on my career, to the neglect of my family and friends.

Is your life filled with things that you enjoy doing? The following situations may point out imbalances in your life. But don't despair; remedies follow!

Too-Much-Career Imbalance

Do you dread the end of a workday because all you seem to do is go home to a lonely apartment? If so, you're working too much. Do you feel indispensable at the office and seem to put in longer hours than your boss? If so, you're working too much.

Vocational-Malaise Imbalance

Have you been taking jobs for the past few years that don't match your abilities, but you can't seem to find that "perfect career"? If so, recognize that this is *not* a dress rehearsal, and you've been waiting for that "perfect job" to fall into your lap for too long. As a result, you feel frustrated most of the time.

No-Special-Someone-To-Love Imbalance

Have you put all your energy into making your career flourish, so that now you're middle-aged and earn a great income, but have no one to share it with?

Have you been heavy most of your life, and although your body gets thinner, you feel like a Neanderthal with the opposite sex? There's no special someone in your life primarily because of the way you feel about yourself.

Same-Old-Routine Imbalance

Do you go out with the *same* friends to the *same* places all the time? If so, you're probably bored because you're not experiencing the excitement created by new interests.

Do you find yourself not looking forward to tomorrow,

thinking, "Is this all there is to life?" If so, you're probably feeling a lack of vitality in your life.

Getting in Balance

If you fall into any of these categories, here are some helpful suggestions. They will involve your taking risks. Be inspired to try some by the familiar wise saying, "Nothing ventured, nothing gained."

If you need to **get that better job**, try some or all of these steps:

1. Set some career goals. If you get confused, meet with a friend who'll help you push through.
2. See a job counselor.
3. Speak to people who enjoy their work, and get some ideas for yourself.
4. Pursue any wild hunches that come up. You'll never know where they might lead.
5. Take stock of your "assets" and know that everything you've done in your life provides useful experiences for whatever new challenges come up.

If you need to **meet new people and develop new interests**, try these ideas:

1. Be adventurous; go to some outlandish place. It could be an event or party. I dare you. If the crowd seems interesting, take some phone numbers.
2. Look at the things you haven't had time for— things that you enjoyed in the past. Now *make* some time. Go to a concert this month, paint one picture, write a poem. It's time for you to make a small commitment by filling out the blanks below:

My Commitment

I,_____, will _____
      (your name)   (activity)
this month.

Appreciate the lovely things around you—flowers, children, birds singing. It will recharge you to take new actions.

To find that special someone, start by acknowledging that you're lovable just the way you are. Affirm that each morning before you leave your house. (I used to wink at myself in a mirror.) No matter what your weight is, don't let your low self-esteem win out. You deserve to have a good life, one that is filled with a beautiful you.

Anticipate the best. Remain optimistic and affirm that "I am an attractive person and my appropriate companion is coming to me now." By all means keep open to the people you meet each day. You never know where that special person may be hiding!

Finding a balance in your life takes time and involves a lot of trial and error. Be patient with yourself and other people. It's worth the effort. After all, you are becoming the most wonderful person you know.

Let's drink a toast (our glasses filled with diet soda, of course): To life! Your *new* life!

11
Your Action Plan

Many of the ideas you'll find in this chapter have already been discussed in this book. It's now time for you to pull it all together. Use the following information as a guideline to start on a positive course of action.

Action 1: Write a Food Plan Each Day

Buy a small notepad and write down what you're going to eat each day. Carry it with you so you can refer to it throughout the day. In that way, you'll *never* be confused as to what to eat.

If your food plan calls for specific amounts of food and you don't trust yourself to take a "normal" portion, weigh each item on a kitchen scale. This doesn't have to be forever—just until you get used to what a normal portion is.

Action 2: Get to Know Your Overeating Patterns

Keep a hunger log for a week. This activity will make you more aware of what types of situations set off your cravings. If you can, write down the experiences as they are happening. At the end of the day, read what you've written, and share it with a friend.

Here's an example of what one page would look like.

Hunger Log

Date _____   Day of the Week _____

Time	Event	Persons Involved

1. _____ _____ _____

   _____ _____ _____

   _____ _____ _____

2. _____ _____ _____

   _____ _____ _____

   _____ _____ _____

3. _____ _____ _____

   _____ _____ _____

   _____ _____ _____

4. _____ _____ _____

   _____ _____ _____

5. _____ _____ _____

   _____ _____ _____

   _____ _____ _____

I noticed the following pattern today regarding my cravings.

_____

_____

_____

_____

_____

When similar situations happen in the future, I will use the following tool to help me get through it (for example, making a phone call to a friend).

_____

_____

_____

_____

After the week is over, you'll probably be more aware of when you're vulnerable to overeating. With this knowledge, list some actions you can take to stay away from excess food.

Vulnerable Times	Supportive Actions
1. *At 10 p.m. before going to sleep.*	*Call a friend.*
2. *At 3 p.m. when the coffee cart comes around.*	*Go to the bathroom and read a section from this book.*
3.	
4.	
5.	

Action 3: Call a Buddy

Designate someone to be your special support person. Check in with him or her at a specific time of day. Share what you've eaten or will eat and any problems you are having. Be sure to talk about the good stuff too! It's nice to have friends who want you to be successful. Listen to your buddy's experiences.

Get in the habit of phoning other people when you're feeling uncomfortable. This will help you break your isolation. Make sure to call other overeaters who have been successful in not overeating. If you stick with the winners, you'll hear a lot of good reasons to stay away from the food.

Be prepared for events where food is served. Work out with your buddy how you're going to handle the occasion. Arm yourself with a specific plan of what you're going to eat. (Call the restaurant before to find out what's going to be served.) Also, make phone calls to other overeaters before, during, and after the meal. And remember, "When in doubt, leave it out!"

Action 4: Join or Start a Support Group Like Overeaters Anonymous

To find an OA meeting, see Appendix D for a central phone number for Overeaters Anonymous. To start your own group, all you need are two other people. Meet with group members at least once a week. When you do, share how you've stayed away from the food during difficult times (that will be a source of strength for everyone). Also, discuss any problems you're having regarding overeating or any other situation in your life.

Set ground rules for sharing. Designate a leader who will call on people and start the discussion. When someone has a problem and seems open to feedback, the leader or a group member can share his or her own experience in dealing with a similar situation. No advice should be given. One person should speak at a time, and no "cross talk" should be allowed.

Action 5: Read Inspirational Literature at Least Once a Day

Carry around some inspirational literature in your bag or briefcase, and read it once a day or more. Choose something that reminds you that other people are overcoming obstacles in their lives. This will inspire you to become successful in your own life. Also, look and listen for success stories in the media about people who are maintaining their weight. Share the stories with your support group.

Action 6: *Reward Yourself*

You're terrific because you've probably endured a lot of pain caused by overeating, and you're ready to find a different way of coping with your life. So reward yourself. Here are some suggestions to help you get started:

- Do something especially nice for yourself each day. You're probably the last person to give yourself credit for things well done. If this is so, try to "stroke" yourself more. Want a creative way of doing this? Splurge! Buy yourself a *toy*, one that's especially for you. Play with it at least twice a day (great for when you're feeling low). This does wonders for the little child in you.

- Make a list at the end of the day of all the nice things that you did for yourself and other people. Take time to think about what you have written.

- Dress your best. Take pride in yourself, no matter what your weight. Bolstering self-esteem starts with *you*.

- Bring nurturing friends into your life, and be willing to avoid binge buddies. Also, develop a relationship with yourself. You're learning to be your own best friend.

- Start simplifying your life. Clean out your refrigerator of unnecessary foods. Simplify your day by avoiding excessive busyness.

- Become aware of your negative mind talk. If you catch yourself thinking phrases like "I'll never be able to _____" or "Other people get all the breaks," *stop* and replace the thought with a positive affirmation: "I *will* be able to _____."

Action 7: Exercise

If you're not already involved in an exercise regimen, make a beginning! Just do five minutes a day to start. Pick an activity that appears in the checklist in Appendix B. Remember that it is important to consult your physician before starting any exercise program.

Action 8: Help Other Overeaters

If the opportunity presents itself, share with other overeaters who are having problems how you've been able to help yourself. To keep what you have, give it away.

Service

Most OAers have received so much from the program that they want to give back what they've gotten, thus maintaining their own recovery and renewing their energy. This takes the form of service, i.e., leading or setting up for meetings, listening to other compulsive overeaters, or just showing up in the group with the desire not to overeat, which strengthens and supports other overeaters.

12
Staying Away from That First Bite

In looking back at my overeating pattern, I see so many times when I took only *one* bite of something I shouldn't have had, and I was soon after eating a lot of things I didn't want to. Most of the time, I wasn't even aware that I was doing this until I got on the scale and saw an increase of five pounds. I would just go off the diet in a small way—even on a dietetic food—and soon after I was off to the races again.

Many OA members have become educated about the seriousness of the first compulsive bite. Let's look at some examples of what that is:

- You've had a fight with your spouse, and dinner has ended. There's no more food left for you to eat on your food plan. To vent your frustrations, you take a bite of an apple. (It wasn't OK for Adam and Eve to do, and it isn't OK for you either!)

- You've been locked up in a meeting with your boss, who's been shooting his mouth off about all the projects that are due Monday. After this session, you feel so frustrated that you go to the company cafeteria and take just *one* bite of a cookie—which, of course, is not part of your food plan.

• You've been strong all day and have stuck to your food plan. But while you are watching TV this evening, your mouth waters as you see a commercial about a new frozen treat. Like a robot, you dash to the refrigerator and eat something you're not supposed to have.

• You're feeling very lonely sleeping by yourself. (The pillow next to you is no substitute for a lover.) Despite these feelings, you fall asleep. However, you wake up in the middle of the night and, half-conscious, head for the fridge and take a bite of something that attracts you.

• You're at a family dinner where the hostess has made a special dish and demands that you taste it. (This taste is not on your food plan.) You think to yourself, "Why not? It's only a harmless little bite," so you acquiesce. After all, you don't want to insult your hostess.

The "menacing" first bite may appear to be an inno-cent action with no further consequences, but it is *not*! For a lot of people, that first bite will always lead to more—if not that hour, then the next day or who knows when? Beware!

If you're not convinced, try taking a little extra of something that you're not supposed to have. See if you can control what you're eating after that. (Give this test a few days.) If you can, then maybe you're not a compul-sive overeater. Many OA members feel similar to alco-holics, who can't take the first drink. The first drink sets up a craving, and most alcoholics are doomed to binge again if they indulge.

Vulnerable Times

When are your vulnerable moments? Are you aware of what triggers your craving for extra food? I wasn't. I'd walk around in a fog, just feeling powerless to control my overeating. I'd be great for a few days on a new diet, and then the cravings would strike. The only thing i could do was succumb to their calling.

However, after many tormenting occurrences, I became more aware of what I was doing and began to arm myself with defenses against that first compulsive bite. For example, I was a night eater—getting up in the middle of the night and walking straight to the refrigerator. What was helpful in stopping that pattern was to keep a diet soda by my bed. When I woke up, I could reach for it immediately. I also kept my "fat picture" taped to the refrigerator as a reminder of what I'd look like with extra pounds on me. When all else failed, I called a friend who didn't mind that I phoned her in the middle of the night. I did that a lot during the early days. All of these actions helped me. This "night eater" is no more!

When Are You Vulnerable to Overeating?

The following instances are when many overeaters report particular vulnerability to reaching for excess food. Check the ones that apply to you. Notice that beneath each scenario there are helpful actions to take. Why not try these alternatives when destructive patterns come up?

_____ I usually overeat late at night.
(Call a food buddy instead.)

_____ As I walk to work, I have a second breakfast. I'm

particularly vulnerable to one bakery en route to the office.
(*Change your walking route and avoid sumptuous food stores.*)

_____ When I go out with friends, I give myself permission to indulge.
(*Tell your friends about your overeating problem and commit to them that you're not going to eat more than your "fair share." This will help you stay honest with your meal. If you hesitate to do this out of fear that your friends will judge you, try to understand that they don't understand about your food problem. But don't let this get in your way. If they're really your friends, they'll support you. If not, maybe it's time to reconsider the friendships.*)

_____ When I wake up in the middle of the night, I go right to the refrigerator.
(*Keep a can of diet soda by your bed table at night.*)

_____ Cocktail parties are a setup for me.
(*Arm yourself with diet soda, coffee, or tea. Know your purpose: to mix with business and social contacts. If you overeat, you probably won't be able to do that.*)

_____ I can't seem to handle eating out in restaurants. I find myself eating too much.
(*Eat at home more often. It's more intimate than dining out anyway. Your source of entertainment doesn't have to be your meals. Turn to other sources: movies, theater, OA meetings.*)

_____ When I'm lonely, I overeat.
(*It's important to take note of what you're missing in your life. Is it a special friend or lover? Remember, food will not take that problem away, and the emptiness will surface again. Overeaters Anonymous provides a fellowship that helps to heal the lonely heart.*)

_____ I lose control during coffee breaks at work.
(*Call a friend and tell him or her that "The Danish is talking to*

me." By sharing that, you won't have to eat it. Keep a notepad by your desk and write down other uncomfortable thoughts that come up.)

Going to Any Lengths

People continue destructive eating behavior because they forget what it's like the "morning after." When they're in the throes of wanting something extra, food seems like an appealing alternative to soothe unpleasant feelings. People block out the harmful effects that usually follow. So when you feel the cravings, it helps to know that they are to be expected, and they *don't* have to win out! The cravings will pass if you go to any length: call a friend and share your discomfort, write down how horrible you'd feel if you gave into the craving, go to your support group or an OA meeting.

▶ ▶ ▶ HELPFUL HINT ◀ ◀ ◀

Write down what your last overeating
episode was like, with *all* its repercussions.
In preparation close your eyes,
visualize the episode, and answer
the following questions:

- What did your body feel like, having taken in all that extra food?

- What were you telling yourself during this episode?

- Did you feel that anyone could help you stop overeating? Describe your feelings.

Carry this paper with you in your wallet. Remember to read it before you take that first bite!

Many OA members can recall the devastation of their food binges and are truly committed to doing whatever it takes to break that cycle. "I had to go to any lengths to stay on my food plan today," says an old-timer to a newcomer. "The program gives me 'tools,' which help me stay away from the food." OA meetings have helped Felicia to remember that no matter what happens in her life, overeating is not an option for her. She goes to at least three OA meetings a week.

"I find meetings are a way of really tanking up on the kind of fuel that's going to allow me to go through the rest of the hours of my day without wanting to eat or having to eat. I don't know that any one tool in and of itself had the effect of making me not want to eat. I think the accumulation of all of them gave me the power to get through my life without reverting to overeating."

This approach boils down to modifying our destructive food habits by reaching out to other people for help. Going to any lengths means a commitment to being alive—to transforming your life into a more meaningful journey.

The following quiz is useful for staying away from that first bite.

Before You Overeat, Consider

Question	Healthy Response OA Member's Answer
1. Will the food help improve the situation that you're confronted with?	No
2. Will you feel nourished after you overeat?	No

3. Do you know that one bite of something you're not supposed to have usually leads to more?   Yes

4. Do you really not care if you gain more weight?   No

5. Are you miserable with the extra weight on your body?   Yes

6. Isn't there another action you could take that would be more positive, like calling a friend or writing how you feel?   Yes

7. Don't you deserve to be good to yourself?   Yes

After you've read the answers to these questions, you probably won't want to overeat. To get some additional support, call a friend and share anything that may have come up as a result of the exercise.

One Day at a Time

One of the things that makes this difficult task easier is the concept of "one day at a time." All we have to do is get through *one* day without overeating. The past is gone, and the future has not come. So the focus is on the moment.

It's easier to live in the present than to plan for a lifetime. The latter seems overwhelming. Making a *daily* commitment to his food plan helps Stanley keep on the straight and narrow.

"Somehow it helps to know that if I really wanted to go out there and binge my brains out, I could do it tomorrow, but I won't do it today."

Here's how Alvin benefits from the concept of one day at a time:

"One day at a time is enormously helpful. I just try to do what I have to for today and let the other problems wait (and they really can!). A lot of people in OA, and certainly myself, want to have all the answers right away. The program teaches me that I don't have to have all the answers; all I have to do is get through this day.

"To people who want to come into Overeaters Anonymous but are afraid that they'll never stick with the program because they've failed at so many diets before, I've said, 'You don't have to make a decision for the rest of your life. Just come to a meeting today. See what it's like; act "as if." ' "

Many members express a deep desire to remain committed to their new way of life. They are willing to face life's challenges without numbing out on excess food. But they weren't always this positive.

"Staying away from that first compulsive bite was a bitch! In the beginning, I acted as if I wanted to. That was enough to get me started on the right track. I didn't have the answers when it came to food and took a 'leap of faith,' trusting that other people did. I did what they suggested and gambled that it would work."

▶ ▶ ▶ HELPFUL HINTS ◀ ◀ ◀

If you're tempted to take that first bite, try this simple delaying exercise. Set a timer for one minute. Tell yourself, "I will not eat for sixty seconds," and *don't*. At the end of this time, you probably won't feel as strongly about the food. If you do, make a

phone call to a friend who will encourage
you not to give in. Repeat this exercise as
many times as you need to throughout the
day. If you're at the office, use the second
hand of your watch as a timer.

Acknowledging the potential power of negative
thoughts is a good practice to get into. These thoughts
can, very cunningly, lead to negative actions such as
overeating. Did you ever glance at what someone else
was eating while in a restaurant and think, "Why can't I
have what's on his plate?" Next time you do that, catch
yourself. If not, you might order another dinner!
Here are some ways of shifting the focus when destructive thoughts surface:

• Mentally say *no* to it: "You may not have my
attention."

• Take a deep breath, and do something productive.

• Call a friend and share your thought. Its power will
be diffused.

• Get in touch with where you are at the moment.
Make a special effort to use your senses—see,
hear, smell the things around you. This will help
quiet your mind.

• Know that dwelling on a destructive thought is the
first step in bringing about a destructive action
(like overeating).

13
Looking to Yourself Rather than Blaming Others

It's so easy to point the finger at other people and absolve yourself of responsibility. It feels good to let out your anger, but after that, what are you left with? When you persist in blaming someone else, it takes an emotional toll on you and can lead to a return to over-eating when you least expect it. Let's take a look at some situations that may sound familiar:

- You're breaking up with an unattentive lover because *it's all his fault!*

- Your parents *never* understand, no matter what you do.

- Your boss is *uncaring* and won't fight for you when raise time rolls around.

These are all examples of blaming other people and not acknowledging your part in the matter. The funny thing about pointing a finger is that when you do it (try it), your thumb is pointing right back at *you*. And the consequence of carrying around resentments is stress, heartache, and loss of physical and emotional energy to move forward in your life.

One way of changing this behavior is to look at what you've done wrong. That's right. In every relationship, *two* people are involved, and at least 50 percent of what goes wrong is your contribution.

It's time to fess up. What relationships in your life are upsetting you? Is there some hurt that you've been holding onto—that's gnawing at you—that's keeping you up at night?

Now let's do the work. Fill out the following chart in order to clarify what your contribution to the problem is. (Use the examples as a guide.)

Person Involved	The Situation	How It Makes Me Feel	My Part in It
1. My boss	He didn't give me a raise.	Angry	I didn't give him my best effort in the last six months.
2. My boyfriend	He forgot my birthday.	Hurt, angry	His mom was in the hospital, and he was preoccupied. I was just

concerned about

_____ _____ _____

_____ _____ _____   _me_.

Now it's your turn to make your list:

_____ _____ _____

_____ _____ _____

_____ _____ _____

_____ _____ _____

_____ _____ _____

_____ _____ _____

_____ _____ _____

   Congratulations. You've just taken a courageous step in your recovery process. By owning your part, you step out of the role of victim, giving up being a person without power who's at the mercy of the world. After all, there are no victims, only volunteers!

Payoffs of Facing Life Squarely

What do we gain by taking responsibility for our actions? Here's a list of the payoffs:

* Self-respect
* Willingness to go forward in your life
* Integrity

- Being part of the imperfect human race
- Looking forward to the day
- Not hiding from your past
- A feeling of lightness, a sense of being guided by something greater than yourself
- The ability to look someone straight in the eye
- A feeling of usefulness to other people
- A sense of excitement

Causes of Blaming Others

What are the underlying causes of our blaming others? They can be summed up very simply by the following five words: anger/hurt feelings, greed, and jealousy.

Let's look at them one at a time. Remember, everyone who's part of the human race has a "darker side."

Anger/Hurt Feelings

We already explored anger and the hurt feelings that usually accompany it. But let's go one step further. The intensity of your feelings about a specific situation is often disproportionate to the situation itself. For example, Heidi is angry at her boyfriend for going away on a fishing trip and not consulting her about this decision. What really irks her is that he made his plans and told her after the fact. This is reminiscent of how Heidi's parents treated her. (They made decisions without involving her.) So her hurt is partially a reaction to the present situation, but the intensity that is evoked is caused by what went on in her past.

Just think about the things in your life that are upsetting you. How many are really caused by what's happening at the moment? The following chart demonstrates that the problems you may be having with people, places, and things are often triggered by your past.

Situation	Present Cause	Memories of the Past
1. My boss tells me one thing and does another	Boss not straight with me.	My father was manipulative like my boss.
2. My wife just criticized me.	Wife's perfectionism.	My mother never thought anything I did was right. My wife is like my mother in that way.

    The point of this exercise is to become more aware of the roots of your anger and blame. If your boss makes you mad, before lashing out at her, take a deeper look and see who you're really angry at—mother, father, or some other person. This may diffuse the intensity of the feeling and give you some distance from which to acknowledge your part in the matter.

Greed

Do you ever have enough of what you want?

Do you ever feel satisfied by your accomplishments?

Do you often look at what someone else has and discount what you have?

Maybe you're always looking for another one of a kind or getting what your friend just got. It never ends.

Greed often takes away from the abundance that is actually in your life at any given moment. It creates discomfort and constant hunger in more ways than one! One solution to this problem is to take a look at all the wonderful things you *have* in your life today.

Jealousy

What fuels your jealousy? When you get right down to it, it's a feeling that you are not enough.

Not quite convinced? Look at the following examples:

- "I'm so jealous that Jill has a boyfriend. I want one."
  Hidden Agenda: "What's wrong with me? I haven't been able to sustain a relationship."

- "Why did John get promoted? I deserve it equally."
  Hidden Agenda: "John seems to expect good things to happen to him. I really feel unworthy of them."

Here's an exercise that will help you with your jealousy. By learning to take the focus off other people and look at what's special about your life, you'll ultimately feel better about yourself. Practice it whenever the "never enoughs" surface. (You may have difficulty doing this because old habits die hard. In that case, ask a friend for help.)

Self-Appreciation

1. What are three things that give you pleasure in your life today?

2. Take stock of an activity that you like to do that you are currently involved in.

3. Tell a friend about a beautiful scene that you experienced this week.

4. Who is a special person in your life today? Why do you consider him or her so?

5. What have you accomplished this year that is a significant achievement in your life? (It doesn't have to be the Medal of Honor!)

6. Make a list of all the people who have reached out to you today.

I was once complaining to Allan, my best friend, "People in my life aren't praising me enough—my boss, family, and friends, etc., etc., etc." I was into the "poor me's."

Allan confronted me on this. He felt that I was being acknowledged left and right, but I couldn't see it because I was wearing my "it's not enough" blinders. He dared me to look for everyone who said something nice to me for one day. He said, "You'll get appreciation from people you'd never expect."

He was right. It started with my doorman giving me a big smile in the morning as I left my apartment building. Then my secretary went out of her way to answer my phone even though she was late for a luncheon appointment. All day, I was surprised at the appreciation I observed.

So the major problem was me. Many people in our

lives acknowledge us all the time, only we don't see it. Moreover, we need to reinforce ourselves. Isn't that a better alternative to waiting for someone to say exactly what you want him or her to say? That might take YEARS!

▶ ▶ ▶ HELPFUL HINTS ◀ ◀ ◀

If you're feeling unappreciated,
try one of these:

- Compliment yourself on a project well done.

- Say something nice to a person close to you. (Remember the Golden Rule.)

- Think of three things that you like about yourself, and keep them in mind throughout the day.

Staying Positive

To avoid blaming others, we need to stay positive. Here's how Sandy maintains an optimistic outlook about her future.

"I came into the program doubting, too smart for my own good. I believed in the worst, but my life has changed dramatically. One of the greatest things that has helped me is a sense of humor. It gives you a perspective on yourself.

"Sometimes I'm about to walk into a grocery store and buy something that I shouldn't. I say to myself, 'Sandy, get a grip on yourself, lighten up—buy a magazine, take a walk, tell a joke, get out of yourself and get interested in someone else. Smile!' I change my direction. I loosen up and lighten up. That's helped me more than anything else."

For Felicia, one of the most positive things that she's done for herself is to be abstinent. When she was a newcomer to OA, members told her, "Just stay abstinent, and everything is going to be OK."

"Just that simple comforting statement kept me optimistic. If I'm abstinent, there's hope that I'll get married someday and fulfill my other dreams, too. That kept motivating me to go forward."

There is no easy answer for how to build your self-esteem. It takes time and a lot of hard work. And if you stop reaching for excess food to fill this "hunger," you'll be way ahead of the game. With support, you can work through anything. Overeaters Anonymous will prove to be a fantastic resource.

Opening Up

You have been given many tools to help you stay away from excess food. The exercises throughout the book have probably increased your awareness as to why you've overeaten—that is, to stuff down your emotional self. In this chapter, you've learned to admit your part in any rift (not easy!). And over and over again, I've tried to drum home the message that you are not alone. There's help from friends and support groups like Overeaters Anonymous.

So what's left? You have what it takes to live a healthy and productive life. It's time to open up and "jump off the cliff." I use that expression because, for many of us, that's what living in a new way feels like. It's very uncomfortable. The analogy of exercising is helpful. If you haven't been doing it for a while, your muscles hurt, but after some practice, you feel fine. It's the same way with opening up and sharing yourself with people; it gets easier the more often you do it.

Don't be surprised that as you start risking in a new way, your old destructive habits begin to kick up. That's a common phenomenon. Expect that, and remember that your heart wants you to move *forward*, even though your body and mind may say *no*. Just keep going despite the pull backward. And if setbacks occur, don't condemn yourself for it—after all, only robots can be perfect!

Here are some small steps to help you open up. Try them, and find out how the tortoise won the race.

1. Tell a trusted friend a secret about yourself that you've been afraid to let him or her know.

2. When someone asks you to do something, answer truthfully—don't just respond the way you think that person wants you to.

3. Do something that you've been avoiding because you've told yourself you didn't have time in your day.

4. Be spontaneous and go with the unexpected. Enjoy an activity that was totally unplanned.

5. Express your love today to one new person. For example, smile at a child, or buy someone a gift.

14
Writing, Literature, Slogans

"The pen is mightier than the sword" the saying goes. Those words are especially true for overeaters.

Many OA members put their problems and life's emotional challenges on paper. These daily practices range from writing a food plan on a small notepad to tallying up an "emotional balance sheet" at the end of the day—an inventory of behavioral pluses and minuses. Writing can also be helpful in remembering what it was like during and after your last food binge. This reminder can aid you in *not* doing it again.

The tool of writing doesn't have to be laborious—you are not in training to be Dostoevski! As with everything else, a little bit of willingness is all you need to begin. Somehow, by writing about what you are feeling at any given moment, you clear the air and diffuse the stress. Alice finds that it helps her identify what's going on in her head.

Sponsors may also give writing assignments to clarify

the various roles that food has played in newcomers' lives. Writing can help with the never-enough syndrome. A gratitude list at the end of the day is a great antidote for overcoming "have nots." As Jackie says, "When I see the things I'm grateful for listed on paper, I can feel thankful for what I *do* have in my life. It is enough; I don't need anything more." (Overeaters tend to always feel "hungry," no matter what's on their plate!)

Sandy takes stock of her day by writing a letter to herself.

> "I write what I liked and what I didn't like about my actions today. I make sure to endorse myself, even though I sometimes don't feel like it.
>
> "For example, today I wrote, 'I showed up at work on time. I worked hard. I had a good attitude. I was honest with my boyfriend, loving but direct. I was abstinent, and I didn't spend compulsively.'
>
> "I also write my negatives: 'I was gossipy at work, which made me uncomfortable. I was obsessed about my weight— my stomach and my thighs. I'm terrified of being fired.' (This has been showing up in my writing for a while.)
>
> "I don't go back and read any of it. I find that writing is a good discipline. It sort of relieves the buildup. It's like flossing your teeth every night. I feel better for doing it."

Natalie is also a letter writer. Writing is a way of purging herself from the painful feelings that come up. For example, she was able to work through a difficult time with her sister, as she describes:

> "I have one sister, and through the years, we've had the poorest of communication with each other. I tried to bridge some kind of gap by writing her a letter and pouring my heart out. I asked her if she would be willing to meet me halfway in terms of trying to be friends as well as sisters.

"Here are a few paragraphs of the letter:

I'm aware of the fact that your personal life has not exactly been the easiest these past months— mine hasn't been easy either. I'm not interested in having a debate, competing with you as to whose is worse. What I have difficulty with is your telling me I'm so unfeeling. That's just another indication of how poorly we've communicated.

I'm sure you have very genuine feelings of your own regarding our relationship. What concerns me is that we still don't communicate or try to understand and love each other. When I have tried to express my hurt, I feel I get back anger instead of compassion and understanding. To defend myself, I cover my hurt by getting angry myself. I cannot recall many instances where there has been caring between us.

I really don't expect you to like or agree with my choices in life. I only ask that you respect that I've selected differently. I do not care to prove to you that my way is better. We walk in different shoes. Somehow, in my heart I have always reserved a special place for you. I know you say you love me because I am your sister, but I only ask that there be peace between us—if not for you and me, then at least for Mom and Pop. I hope we can work this out.

"My sister wrote me a letter explaining her feelings and how she felt about me when we were growing up and now. We came to peace. She's very different from me. We have extremely different lifestyles. She lives in the suburbs, I live in the city. I'm divorced, and she's married with three children. At forty-five, she went back to college, and I graduated over twenty years ago. I guess she stopped trying to be my mother, and we were able to find a common ground."

▶ ▶ ▶ HELPFUL HINTS ◀ ◀ ◀

Here are some ways writing can work for you:

- Write down your food plan each day on a small notepad. Keep it with you and refer to it before meals. (You can see I'm big on this one—I've mentioned it several times.)

- Take stock of your emotional thermostat. If something is bothering you, write about it. The pen will help you work through your feelings.

- Write letters to yourself or a person you're having difficulty with. Describe your feelings. Remember, you don't have to mail these letters.

- Make a Gratitude List at the end of the day, including all that you appreciate. This exercise will help you stay optimistic about your life.

- Keep a record of Daily Checks and Balances (the balance sheet referred to at the beginning of this chapter). Make a list with these two column headings and be sure to fill it out each day:

Day *Monday*

Could Do Better	Great Job
1. *More courteous to my boss.*	*Helped my sister.*
2. *Less gossipy at work.*	*Friendly to neighbors.*
3.	
4.	

Take a look at the things you could have improved on today, i.e., *not courteous to my boss* or *gossiping at work*. Also make sure to fill up the other side of the sheet—*warm and friendly to my neighbors, helped my sister with clothes shopping*. You're looking for a balance here, the good as well as the bad.

Literature

When all else fails, reading something inspiring helps! OA publishes pamphlets and a few books that give insightful information about compulsive overeating. Also, many overeaters use the "Big Book" of Alcoholics Anonymous for insight into addiction and the 12 Steps of Recovery. (Call AA World Services for more information.) This and other enlightening material come in handy when you're waiting in a grocery line and want to eat everything that's in your neighbor's shopping cart.

At night, when the cravings start and you want to attack the refrigerator . . . *don't*. Instead, turn to a story about someone who is recovering. It will fill your "soul hunger" better than your favorite candy bar ever could. Sandy reads from two small books each morning before she goes to work.

> "*One of these meditation books I started reading eight years ago when I first entered the program. I supplement it with another little book. Throughout my workday, I try to remember what the readings suggest. It's a way of getting myself on a positive track. I remember that there's help available if I am just willing to reach out for it.*
>
> "*Right now, my business is in turmoil. People on the job are afraid of layoffs and firings. The readings are especially helpful. I read everything twice so it really sticks!*"

▶ ▶ ▶ HELPFUL HINTS ◀ ◀ ◀

• Carry around in your purse or pocket something

inspiring to read during the day when the munchies strike.

* Go to a bookstore and search the racks for a new book with some type of "soul food" in it.

Slogans

OA members have simple sayings that are packed with wisdom. They have helped many overeaters who live in a fast-track world sort out their priorities. Why not make up some of your own, such as:

* "The food won't help" (to be used in any situation)

* "What are my priorities?" (when you feel overwhelmed)

* "I'm a wonderful person" (when you're feeling low)

* "There are no failures, just slow successes" (for acknowledging your actions, however imperfect they may be)

Repeat these silently to yourself, and see if you don't feel better.

15
Addressing the New You

It wasn't easy for me to break old habits. Many times I would lose the weight, stay there for a while, and gain it back, sometimes gradually, sometimes right away. But it would always come back. This was a "safe" pattern for me. The fat buffered me from the world; I kept a comfortable distance between myself and people. Changing my lifestyle and becoming thin often involved a lot of emotional discomfort, but it was worth the struggle.

"Thin Shock"

When I was thin, I was afraid of the skinny person who appeared in the mirror. Who was that attractive woman walking down the street? Men were flirting with me at parties. How could I cope with being so visible? My boundaries were being invaded. I wore my fat as a source of protection—without it, I felt vulnerable, out of control over my new life.

Other overeaters have talked about having similar problems when they get down to maintenance weight. Their concern is not only what foods to take back, but how to become more comfortable in their "new skin"— you know, the "I look so good, I can't handle it" syndrome. OA members support each other to accept their attractiveness and everything that goes along with it. People are encouraged to move ahead in their lives.

Self-acceptance involves a gradual process, and honesty is a necessary component of it. You must be willing to let someone else know the truth about how you feel. It eventually becomes easier to accept the new you. It's similar to what happens when you break in new shoes. At first they feel stiff and tight, but gradually you grow into them.

Besides the physical changes, you must come to terms with the emotions that come up as a result of your being an active participant in life. You'll probably find that your relationships will be in a state of flux. Just a few of the questions that you will be confronted with are: How do I face someone who's not treating me well? How do I tell him or her *no*, especially when I've always said *yes*? How do I put myself first? I usually come last! It takes time to work these issues through. Overeaters Anonymous is a terrific support.

Growing involves a lot of discomfort, and sometimes the lure of food seems tempting. But OA members will remind you that overeating isn't a viable option. You still have to deal with the same problems after you finish a food binge. Nothing goes away.

The concept of one day at a time helps you handle each problem as it comes up. One old-timer says, "As long as I keep focused on today, I can manage my life." You face situations from telling your boss that you need more help in the office to letting your husband know that he's making dinner for the kids tonight because you're going to an OA meeting. In Overeaters Anonymous, you can work out any challenge that may arise. Someone is always available to talk things over.

Facing the New You

What are some of the fears you may have about experiencing a new you? Go through the following list, and see which ones apply:

- I'll never be able to maintain a thin body.

- I'm afraid of my sexual feelings.

- How will I be able to cope with all the attention I'll get from people? I'm used to hiding.

- I've never put myself first. It will create a lot of waves with my family and friends.

- How will I handle it all—I have more friends and responsibilities than I've ever had before!

- Will some of my relationships end?

- Once I get a taste of my new self-esteem, I'll never be able to go back to old habits.

- I'll be visible and have to become more responsible for my life.

- I don't want to face the feelings that will come up. How will I be able to cope with them?

- I'm so frightened to get close to other people.

You probably have many of these concerns. But it's worth it to face them head on. And with a little help from friends or a professional, you can tackle them one by one.

Some overeaters seem to share a common pattern: once they get close to goal weight, they become afraid and slip, going back to their destructive food patterns. You *don't* have to do this, and you *can* learn from their mistakes. OA will give you the added support to face life's challenges in a new way. But you'll have to give up your false pride that you're so much different from everyone else! If you do this, the rewards are tremendous. Just look at a few:

• A more fulfilled life

• Loving relationships

• Self-esteem

• A leaner body

• Looking forward to each day

• A more creative life at work and at home

• Feeling as if there's a purpose to your life

• Enjoying yourself

• Enhancing the lives of other people

• Truly loving yourself

Why not give it a try? The people who care about you want you to.

Reaping the Rewards

When you reach your goal and trim down to size, it isn't easy coping with the new you. You're confronted with core issues like asserting yourself to get your needs met and learning to say *no* despite the guilt that may surface. No easy task! Practicing this new behavior can feel very uncomfortable.

Not only is this difficult for you, but it takes a lot of adjusting for your friends, family, and co-workers too. Some people will be upset with the new, assertive you.

Eating buddies may resent what they see as your betrayal. A lot of people may have to change the way they've been relating to you.

What keeps us pressing forward, despite the discomfort, is that we begin to reap the rewards of making healthier choices for ourselves, namely, self-esteem and peace of mind.

Choices

Life without overeating boils down to the realization that we have choices. When I was overeating, life seemed to be one empty tunnel of "have to's"; my free will went out the window. This type of existence was very safe. I knew where I was going—the same place I had been yesterday—and next week would be the same as today! So I didn't have to take any risks, because I wasn't moving forward in my life.

In putting down excess food, we choose life! Staying away from excess food allows me to face life's rewards and challenges, and living in this transformed way is very scary at times. I make many choices each day, some of which advance me and a few that set me back. I'm living life imperfectly, but I'm *showing up*. I have energy to do all sorts of things.

When I started experiencing all this good stuff, I found myself getting impatient and melancholic. I wanted everything that I had previously missed out on *now*! I had to learn that I would receive things in their right time, and not on my schedule. For example, I felt ready to get remarried and meet someone special for a year, yet nothing happened. I guess I wasn't as ready as I thought. I met my new husband two years later.

Regretting is an energy drain. "If only I had these good feelings a few years ago, I could have accomplished so much more." This type of thinking was a booby trap for me, draining my energy and vitality. I realized that I can't change how I've been throughout

my life, but I can share what I've learned with other
people who may need some help from me.

Creating a Terrific Life Today
What's the secret to having a terrific life? You guessed
it: not turning to food for comfort. Food is not my best
friend, lover, or confidant today.

Food Is:	Food Is Not:
Sustenance	A friend
Nourishment	My confidant
Something to be enjoyed	My Saturday-night date

I want the quality of my life to be upgraded, and I am
willing to do whatever it takes to make it happen. My
self-esteem increased as I was able to let people help
me.

Here are some other ways I created more joy in my
life:

- I recommitted myself to not overeating each day.

- I made it my business each day to acknowledge
  something positive that I did for myself.

- I accepted a compliment if it was given to me.

- I took good physical care of myself through efforts
  such as dressing well.

- I allowed myself to be my own best friend, trying
  to change my "negative tapes" to positive ones.

- I put myself in "intensive care." I accepted that for
  a time I would feel empty and tried not to
  substitute excessive activity (workaholism) to fill
  the void.

- I was very gentle with myself and began to nurture

myself. Having loving friends helped me to learn this new behavior.

I hope the examples will give you some ideas for your own life. The truth is that I really didn't feel that I "deserved" all the good things in life (even though I said I did). I also didn't realize my true value as a person or the impact I had on other people. Do you realize the impact *you* have on people?

Despite what you may think, you do make a difference in the world, no matter what your weight. The more I hid behind my fat and thought, "No one would really miss me if I weren't there," the more depressed I became. You see, I made a difference but didn't know it, and *you do, too!*

Keep these truths in mind:

• People *do* want to hear your thoughts on things.

• If you're not present when you've said you'll be somewhere, the other person will be concerned.

• When you're with a group of people, no one but you is thinking how fat you are. They probably have more important things to think about.

The most important realization I had throughout the years is that, as overeaters, we are all closely interconnected. Even though our histories are different, we feel, think, live, and die. What makes my life's journey interesting is all the wonderful people I've met along the way. Our greatest defeats (bulges, excess weight, being out of control with food) can become our greatest asset, because they teach us things we can use to help other people.

In breaking through and overcoming our destructive overeating patterns, we have an opportunity to share our strength, hope, and experience with other people. Through a crippling disorder, we learn how to be vulnerable. Like the ripples from a tiny pebble thrown into a lake, let your tears, laughter, and growth extend outward to touch other overeaters. In this way, we are able to shed our isolationist skin and become vulnerable again. We no longer need the fat to hide behind; we are whole and complete on our own.

Appendix A: Nutrition Review

This information has been adapted from *Nutrition and Your Health: Dietary Guidelines for Americans*, 2nd ed., Home and Garden Bulletin No. 232 (U. S. Department of Agriculture, U.S. Department of Health and Human Services, 1985). There is loads of information that you can write away for.

To assure yourself an adequate diet, eat a variety of foods daily in adequate amounts, including selections from the following:

- Fruits

- Vegetables

- Whole-grain and enriched breads, cereals, and other products made from grains

- Milk, cheese, yogurt, and other products made from milk

- Meats, poultry, fish, eggs, and dry beans and peas

To lose weight, eat a variety of foods that are low in calories and high in nutrients:

- Eat more fruits, vegetables, and whole grains
- Eat less fat and fatty foods
- Eat less sugar and sweets
- Drink fewer alcoholic beverages
- Increase your physical activity

To avoid too much fat, saturated fat, and cholesterol, follow these guidelines:

- Choose lean meat, fish, poultry, and dry beans and peas as protein sources
- Use skim milk or low-fat milk and milk products
- Moderate your use of egg yolks and organ meats
- Limit your intake of fats and oils, especially those high in saturated fats, such as butter, cream, lard, heavily hydrogenated fats (some margarines), shortenings, and foods containing palm and coconut oils
- Trim fat off meats
- Broil, bake, or boil rather than fry
- Moderate your use of foods that contain fat, such as breaded and deep-fried foods
- Read labels carefully to determine both amount and type of fat present in foods

To eat more starch and fiber, follow these guidelines:

- Choose foods that are good sources of fiber and starch, such as whole-grain breads and cereals, fruits, vegetables, and dry beans and peas

- Substitute starchy foods for those that have large amounts of fats and sugars

To avoid too much sugar, follow these suggestions:

- Use less of all sugars and foods containing large amounts of sugars, including white sugar, brown sugar, raw sugar, honey, and syrups. Examples include soft drinks, candies, cakes, and cookies.

- Remember, *how often* you eat sugar and sugar-containing food is as important to the health of your teeth as *how much* sugar you eat. It will help to avoid eating sweets between meals.

- Read food labels for clues on sugar content. If the words *sugar, sucrose, glucose, maltose, dextrose, lactose, fructose,* or *syrups* appear first, then there is a large amount of sugar.

- Select fresh fruits or fruits processed without syrup or with light, rather than heavy, syrup

Appendix B:
Exercise Helpers

I don't need to tell you that exercise is important. You most likely know that about exercise, but doing it is another matter. So I'll give you a few pointers to help you get started toning different parts of your body.

How do you get yourself to exercise? That's the rub, isn't it? There's one sure way *not* to—that is to expect too much of yourself too soon and fall short of your goals. Instead, take small actions, which you can increase once you've begun. Of course, if you already have an exercise regimen, bravo!

Hate your body? It's all you've got right now, so remember these helpful hints:

- Be compassionate with yourself. Blaming yourself for your excess weight will get you nowhere—in fact, it might lead to your becoming so frustrated that you'll want to overeat again. Be gentle with your body as you exercise. Love it into shape.

- Select an exercise activity, and make a beginning (if only for five minutes each day). You'll increase your routine with time. Check with your physician before starting any exercise program. Here are some suggested activities:

  - Walking

  - Jogging

  - Running

  - Swimming

  - Raquetball

  - Tennis

  - Karate

  - Working out at a gym

  - Aerobic dancing

  - Popular dancing

  - Baseball

  - Volleyball

  - Roller skating

  - Yoga

- Think about buying an exercise book. Browse in the library or bookstore, and see what appeals to you. Buy or check out one or two books that look interesting. A regular program makes it easier for some people to get started.

Another way of looking at your situation is that you can't change the damage that's been done already. However, you can learn from this experience by keeping your memory fresh. The next time something delicious calls, remember how difficult it is *now* to lose weight. This will help you stay away from the food.

By the way, for many people binge weight comes off easily if you exercise and cut down your food. And whatever you do, *don't weigh yourself more than once a month*. Anything more is just a setup for you to get discouraged.

Appendix C:
Suggested Readings

Alcoholics Anonymous: The Story of How Many Thousands of Men and Women Have Recovered from Alcoholism, 3rd ed. New York: A. A. World Services Inc., 1976.

B., Bill. *Compulsive Overeater*. Minneapolis, Minn.: Comp-Care Publications, 1981.

B., Bill. *Maintenance*. Minneapolis, Minn.: CompCare Publications, 1986.

Food for Thought: Daily Meditations. Minneapolis, Minn.: Hazelden Foundation, 1980.

For Today. Torrance, Calif.: Overeaters Anonymous, 1982.

Hollis, Judi. *Fat Is a Family Affair*. Center City, Minn.: Hazelden Foundation, 1985.

Lerner, H. *Stress Breakers*. Minneapolis, Minn.: CompCare Publications, 1985.

Listen to the Hunger. Center City, Minn.: Hazelden Foundation, 1987.

12 Steps and 12 Traditions. New York: A. A. World Services Inc., 1952.

Appendix D:
Additional Sources of Information

For additional information on Overeaters Anonymous, consult your local telephone directory under Overeaters Anonymous, or call (213) 542-8363.

For additional information on nutrition, write to:

The Human Nutrition Information Service
U. S. Department of Agriculture
Room 360
6505 Belcrest Road
Hyattsville, MD 20782

You might also contact state and local public health departments and state or local medical societies.